P E A K
PERFORMANCE

BODY & MIND

T0273742

Dr. Scott W. Donkin
& Dr. Gérard Meyer

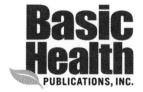

Basic
Health
PUBLICATIONS, INC.

The information contained in this book is based upon the research and personal and professional experiences of the authors. It is not intended as a substitute for consulting with your physician or other healthcare provider. Any attempt to diagnose and treat an illness should be done under the direction of a healthcare professional.

The publisher does not advocate the use of any particular healthcare protocol but believes the information in this book should be available to the public. The publisher and authors are not responsible for any adverse effects or consequences resulting from the use of the suggestions, preparations, or procedures discussed in this book. Should the reader have any questions concerning the appropriateness of any procedures or preparation mentioned, the authors and the publisher strongly suggest consulting a professional healthcare advisor.

Basic Health Publications, Inc.
8200 Boulevard East
North Bergen, NJ 07047
1-201-868-8336

Library of Congress Cataloging-in-Publication Data
Donkin, Scott W.
    Peak performance : body & mind / Scott W. Donkin and Gérard Meyer.
        p. ; cm.
Includes bibliographical references and index.
    ISBN 1-59120-014-8
    1. Human mechanics. 2. Health. 3. Human engineering.
    [DNLM: 1. Mind-Body Relations (Metaphysics)—Popular Works.
2. Health Promotion—methods—Popular Works. 3. Holistic Health—Popular
Works. WB 880 D684p 2002] I. Meyer, Gérard, 1947– II. Title.
    QP301 .D59   2002
    613—dc21

                                            200200667

Editor: Roberta W. Waddell
Typesetter/Book design: Gary A. Rosenberg
Cover design: The Great American Art Company

Printed in the United States of America

10 9 8 7 6 5 4 3 2 1

CONTENTS

This book is dedicated to my family, friends,
and colleagues who have supported or challenged me.
You have all made this book better.

This dedication also extends to my patients,
who have always been my most prolific teachers,
and to my sources of *Inspiration*.

—*Dr. Scott W. Donkin*

This book is dedicated to two important groups
motivating my life:

My loving family and friends,
because they never doubted my ability
to always create what I dreamed of,
and because they support me unconditionally,
through my madness, in my desire to improve the world.

And the doubtful, negative people
that I enjoy challenging so much
by proving that nothing is more powerful
than the spark of an idea received from The Higher Power,
which can succeed in changing the world for the better.

—*Dr. Gérard Meyer*

FOREWORD

"SIT UP STRAIGHT!"

No matter what your generation, you heard it from your parents like a mantra. Not that you listened. It was one of those phrases it was easy to obey for about five seconds and then ignore as if you never heard it.

But there is a lot of ancient wisdom in those three words. Your parents probably didn't take time or have enough information to explain it (and, of course, you weren't listening anyway), but sitting up straight is vital to keeping your body working properly.

One of the keys that I have learned in my years of practicing medicine, first in traditional medicine, and later using alternative treatments, is that everything in your body is connected to everything else. No disorder affects just one part. That maxim is nowhere more evident than when talking about ailments caused by lack of skeletal support. When we don't work with the way our bodies are made and take advantage of the strength of our skeletons, it puts undue stress on muscles, joints, tendons, and especially nerves. That causes disruptions in nerve communication, pain, restricted movement, and restricted blood flow. Since none of that feels good, your breathing becomes shallow, limiting the oxygen supplied to your brain, and sending you into a depressed emotional state. The restricted flow of blood, oxygen, and nerve impulses takes the vital energy from your whole body and sets you up for increased oxidative stress, which attacks your vital organs and can cause heart disease, cancer, and a host of other degenerative diseases.

The way to prevent all of that from happening is contained in that seed, "Sit up straight." It is not a matter of how it looks; it's a matter of what it does to your health. In this book, Drs. Donkin and Meyer help us to understand just what it means to sit up straight, what happens when we don't, and how we can solve the problems that are caused by making our bodies adjust to our environment rather than adjusting our environment to work with our bodies. It's simple practical advice containing that uncommon quality of common sense.

Most of us have, at one point, known someone who was living in an intolerable situation—with an abusive spouse, a disobedient child, a manipulative partner, etc. It is easy for us to see from the outside what the problem is and see that our friend could solve it by just changing the way he or she fits into the situation. But our friend doesn't have the perspective to see just how messed up the situation is or how ridiculous the accommodations he or she has made to survive in it are. People in these situations see themselves as victims who are powerless, yet the truth is that they could change the situation very simply.

Drs. Donkin and Meyer give us guidance to look at the intolerable situation we often live with in respect to what we do to our bodies. We may live with intolerable pain, but they help us look at what we are doing to cause that pain. They help us look at what we are doing to our bodies when we sleep, when we work, when we exercise, when we play, when we do yard work, even when we sneeze, and show us how to find better ways to avoid pain.

Most important, as you read this book you will see quite clearly that your health is in your hands. You have the power to control your health, and it is solely your responsibility to do so. Most of the problems physicians treat are a result of bad habits—those actions that we have ingrained in our bodies over time through repetition. Smoking is one and it has its consequences; slouching, overreaching, improper lifting, and bad sleeping position are others and they have their consequences. The good news is that changing your pillow is a lot easier than quitting smoking—so is rearranging your workspace or developing good posture. The point is that the only way to correct bad habits is to replace them with good ones. It is all up to you.

You have the choice to work with your body—in ways that match the way your body is built—or you can force your body into all kinds of convoluted positions that cause pain and disease and be miserable. If you choose the first, you can enjoy a long, happy, and active life. If you choose the second, you have already ceased to truly live and no matter how long you keep breathing, you can't enjoy what you have.

Change your habits; change your destiny. It's all up to you.

—*James Balch, M.D.*

PREFACE

Two Different Paths to the Same Destination

A Personal Message from Dr. Gérard Meyer

I can easily recall the thunderous, compressive explosion of metal and shattering windshield glass the moment my car, traveling at 75 miles per hour, slammed into the front of a cargo truck speeding toward me at 60 miles per hour. Horrified bystanders were afraid to come near me for fear that my car, with leaking gasoline, would explode. As I pulled myself out and pushed away from the wreckage, there were unforgettable sounds of chaos and smells of danger. The doctors in the emergency room diagnosed and treated my numerous injuries, which included several broken teeth, facial bone fractures, a broken jaw, three broken ribs, a broken kneecap exposed by a large bleeding gash over my right knee, and substantial spinal damage. Fortunately, I was the only person injured. But my car, the truck, and most of its load were destroyed.

The moment of the accident clearly altered my life, but the words "moment" and "accident" are very misleading. First, many factors led up to that moment and the event really was no accident. It was, instead, a series of events that predictably caused this outcome. In recalling the evolution of this accident, it is important to note that just prior to it: 1) I was a young, ambitious businessman in Paris and had, for several days, been intensely working on a project to sell to another company. 2) The preparation for my upcoming meeting had been very stressful and exhausting. 3) Because I had been working so hard on this project, I had neglected my tires, which were becoming very worn. 4) I recognized that they were wearing down, but decided not to change them because I thought I was too busy, and I also wanted to save money by buying new ones at a later date.

5) I woke up a little bit late for my plane trip to this important meeting so I rushed to get ready. 6) I discovered that the shirt I wanted to wear was not washed and pressed, so I was upset and had an argument with my wife. 7) Wearing my unwashed, unpressed shirt, I left by slamming the door and walked briskly across the yard, still soaked from the early morning dew, and sped out toward the airport along the wet streets and highways. 8) The car ahead was traveling too slowly for me so I decided to pass as fast as I could by accelerating around it in the oncoming lane. 9) This car then sped up so I had to go faster to get around because I was in too big a hurry to slow down and pull back behind it. 10) At that point, the speeding truck appeared in front of me. 11) I slammed on the brakes and oversteered to avoid him but headed, skidding, right for his front bumper anyway, and then there was the awful impact.

I realize now how many factors led to this accident and know that if I had recognized what was happening and had altered even one of the events in the series just described, the accident would never have happened. For example: 1) If I had paid more attention to proper vehicle maintenance, and had gotten new tires, my steering on the slick highways could have kept me from having the impact. 2) If I hadn't been so upset, I would not have made the unwise decision to pass the car ahead of me. 3) If I hadn't been so stressed and fatigued, my reaction time would have been better. 4) If I hadn't been so preoccupied with making the flight and having a great meeting, I would have recognized the danger I was heading toward. 5) If I had been trained to drive and steer on wet, slippery roads, I would have known to reduce my speed, properly apply the brakes, and steer away from danger. 6) If I had left five minutes earlier, I never would have been behind that slow car in the first place. (I might have been behind another one, but I probably wouldn't have tried to pass.)

The medical definition of an accident is an often predictable series of events that leads to an injury. I believe this is true of all accidents, and the accident I just described illustrates this phenomenon. That moment marked a change in my life. After it, I decided to create (sooner or later— a quarter of a century later in this case) a system in which it is possible to attain transportation safety by training drivers to have increased awareness of high-risk events and have increased driving skills, especially in hazardous conditions, in order to actually prevent accidents.

The series of events leading to an accident are similar to the habits that lead to a premature breakdown of the physical body. There is a predictable series of events that occur in your daily habits which determine whether you will enjoy good physical health and longevity, or will experience gradual physical decline. Every day you make thousands of subconscious, habitual, and conscious choices that collectively shape your destiny. Most simple actions or inactions bypass your awareness and, therefore, leave you feeling as though you are not in control. However, becoming aware of these actions and habits, and systematically improving them to suit your needs and long-term goals is quite possible and practical. The result is that you are much more in control than you previously thought. And, by the time you finish this book, the choice of how you will live out your life will be yours to make.

A Personal Message from Dr. Scott Donkin

Peak Performance: Body & Mind has evolved from an expanded form of my first book, *Sitting on the Job,* into a comprehensive yet practical guide to developing your own peak performance, body and mind. Peak performance in a motor vehicle, for example, occurs when all systems and their components are functioning at their optimum levels and are in concert with one another. The vehicle operates most effectively and safely in these circumstances, which enable it to have a much longer, useful life.

As humans, peak performance occurs when our own systems are working in unison and our mind's awareness of the body and its surroundings enables heightened concentration, anticipation, and reflex action. Achieving peak performance is different from expending maximum effort. Maximum effort in physical conditioning is used to improve the physical condition so that peak performance can occur at a more efficient level. But maximum effort cannot be sustained, and, if performed too often without careful conditioning management, it can actually lead to injury and a breakdown of the body and mind.

Peak performance, on the other hand, is a very desirable and often exhilarating state. In addition, as we describe in this book, it is a sustainable state that has many far-reaching benefits. This book is designed to give you a systematic approach to living your life at a much higher level of comfort, satisfaction, and accomplishment. You will learn the causes of gradual injury, how they differ from the causes of sudden injury, and the special methods needed to prevent their occurrence. The concepts applied here are fundamentally the same as those used to prevent motor vehicle accidents.

Optimizing the use and condition of your body will increase your resistance to injury and fatigue, decrease the cumulative negative impact of stress, and improve sleep habits, thereby reducing the onset and effects of sleep deprivation. The positive result of conditioning your body to achieve peak performance is a greater sense of alertness, an increased feeling of accomplishment, and a healthier, injury-free body and mind.

I will always remember my first glimpse of the connection between physical health, prevention, and safety, and motor vehicle health, prevention, and safety. Dr. Gérard Meyer, then President and CEO of The Carnegie Mellon Driver Training and Safety Institute (CM-DTSI), had just picked me up at the Pittsburgh airport. We were traveling to the institute campus he was just beginning to develop. Dr. Meyer was explaining his theory and vision of accident prevention with motor vehicles. He described, in vivid detail, his approach to creating a system of training whereby a driver (or any other worker with a mobile job) will be traveling, first in a truck, then in other vehicles, which are well-maintained and operating at expected performance levels, and in which the driver is sitting correctly, with the gearshift, steering wheel, mirrors, and other controls appropriately positioned. This driver is in the optimum state of mind and physical condition to produce an acute state of awareness and uses his or her senses to anticipate trouble and either avoid or minimize danger's impact. But, Dr. Meyer quickly added, since hazardous driving conditions, heavy traffic, and other stresses occur regularly on the road, the driver must be trained in the exact handling of the vehicle and must be able to practice driving in hazardous conditions. Only with this exacting training can the driver respond with the swift and correct response that is necessary, and that can be recalled automatically, when the need presents itself.

This same exact principle applies to the drivers' uses of their own bodies. They must be trained and practiced in the proper, practical use and handling of their bodies, even under less than ideal conditions, so they can avoid the negative impact of a dangerous situation. Health and safety are directly connected. A healthy, well-balanced body performs better. A healthy, well-balanced mind performs better. The first step in safety must be to recognize the tie between the two.

The goal is to create a sustainable safety system that actually prevents transportation accidents and physical injuries. The Bio Ergonomic Safety Theory (B.E.S.T.), created by Dr. Meyer, is the comprehensive approach to this (although the theory itself is not fully explained here, many of its fundamental concepts are represented in this text).

In order to master any given task, such as truck driving, an intimate knowledge of, and trained skill in the use, handling, and care of the truck in all conditions and circumstances is necessary. Since truck driving is a whole body and mind activity, it also follows that an intimate knowledge, and trained skill level in the use, handling, and care of the body, in all conditions and circumstances, is necessary.

Mastering the art of driving well requires mastering the use of both the truck and the body so, in this book, we explain and elaborate on merging the concepts of truck and body performance to ensure that these two separate and distinct systems can perform as one in a sustainable system of safety and success. Even for those who are not professional drivers, Dr. Meyer's method is an ideal way to learn about the use and care of their own bodies so that gradual wear and tear can be minimized and a long, physically satisfying life can be achieved.

Part I deals with the fundamentals of achieving a perfect fit for our bodies, focusing on seven basic principles—balance, form, flow, time, repetition, force, and flexibility—and our anatomy as we age. Part II explains how to apply the fundamentals we have outlined to your life, and in Part III, we discuss prevention and total body management. Throughout, we will use the interaction between human and machine to illustrate the similarities and differences between the systems, and to fully explain how you and others can improve yourselves in surprisingly simple ways you may not previously have thought possible.

ACKNOWLEDGMENTS

Dr. Scott W. Donkin

This book took several forms over the last six years and many people have helped me through its evolution. My wife, Mary Pat, and my children, Elizabeth and Peter, have been very patient with me and have endured a lot, not always knowing in what direction I was heading with this work, or when it would finally be completed.

Likewise, I am grateful to my partner, Dr. David Lauer, and his wife, Kelly, who graciously put up with my distractions and the time I spent away from our practice during this project. Dr. Heather Elton, Dru Fogerty, and the rest of our staff, including Paul, Angie, Ashlie, Holly, Jacque, Jami, Jamie, and Tori have been most accepting of my attention to this project and of the difficulties I have had managing my time.

I credit several great philosophers of the past, men such as Socrates, Aristotle, and Plato, with shaping my understanding of the forms in the world around me and providing me with a method for questioning the world in order to help make it better. Their work lives on.

I thank Michael Gelb for creating multimedia programs that taught me how to capture thoughts and ideas, write them down, and organize them in a cohesive way.

Jan Kelly-Weinberg was instrumental in editing and combining the diverse sections of this book in a way that balanced the fundamental concepts with practical application. Sandy Wendel also applied her expertise to vastly improve the earliest version. Mark Hirschfeld was encouraging throughout the evolution of this book, and helped formulate the final version of the important Peak Performance Self-Evaluation Test in Appendix

A. Nicki Nix and David Allee used their artistic abilities to clarify the illustrations and offer objective feedback on key sections of this book.

Dr. Ritch Miller, Dr. Louis Sportelli, Dr. Jerry McAndrews, Pam Wessel, and Dr. Joseph Sweere, a lifetime mentor, read sections of this book and offered their own diverse perspectives on its content, which helped to clarify key concepts.

Dr. Gérard Meyer lifted the quality and usefulness of this book to a much higher level with his contributions, including his conception of the Peak Performance Self-Evaluation Test. He is truly a remarkable man whose dedication and hard work in researching and developing better ways to train drivers will ultimately allow us all to share the highways and streets around the world more safely.

Finally, I would like to say thanks to Bobby Waddell, whose final editing and literal nature made the book flow better than anyone else could have, and to Norman Goldfind, who had the vision and resolve to publish this book.

Dr. Gérard Meyer

I wish to acknowledge my family, including my two daughters Nathalie and Stephanie, my six grandchildren and two more on the way, my friends, and all the exceptional people I have been fortunate enough to be associated with, some of them accidentally, though never without a purpose.

I started this adventure with the idea of collaborating on a book with the well-known author and chiropractor Dr. Scott W. Donkin. My dream was to combine the professional toolboxes of two different kinds of healers to achieve better minds and bodies, on my end using the knowledge I was privileged to acquire in Europe from the famous pioneer in bio-ergonomics, my professor and mentor, Dr. Alain Wisner. In his long and rich career, Dr. Wisner has been devoted to advancing the understanding of human factors in our contemporary society, and he has been instrumental in inspiring me and others like me to improve future working and living environments.

I could never have succeeded in creating the Carnegie Mellon Driver Training and Safety Institute (CM-DTSI) without the help and trust of my friend, the late Dr. Paul Christiano, then Provost of Carnegie Mellon University. He allowed me to create a state-of-the-art living laboratory where

I could apply all safety aspects in everyday life to motor vehicle operators. At CM-DTSI in America, and with our European network of partners, we conducted research and training on how to prevent accidents with workers who are operating mobile job stations.

I wish to acknowledge the support of my team at CM-DTSI/Pittsburgh in helping me achieve my holistic approach to safety, which culminated in the development of The Bio-Ergonomic Safety Theory (B.E.S.T), and most particularly the enthusiastic advice of my friend and colleague Dr. Renee Forne.

I also want to acknowledge my coauthor, Dr. Scott Donkin. We became more than just coauthors and partners. We now are great friends and we have learned a lot from each other. He cured me of an old, chronic back pain (the result of a car accident), in the process giving me the great gift of a better and happier life. Thanks to his healing skills, I feel much more energetic, even young enough to pull the world by the tail. For whatever forces of destiny put us together, I have to give thanks, not only for giving us the chance to synergistically combine our experiences, but also for giving us the privilege of sharing a new approach with you, one which we hope will significantly improve your daily life.

We are only the messengers, however. We want you to consider *yourself* a priority! Use the advice and information we are providing in this book and let it motivate you to become a *work in progress* for your own better, brighter future.

INTRODUCTION

First, try to visualize an overhead view of motor vehicles gridlocked on the Los Angeles freeways, and then visualize, if you can, an alternate view of masses of people in a crowded airport or train station.

The crowded roadways are made up of individual motor vehicles that all have their own control systems and individual destinations. Similarly, the crowded transportation terminals are made up of individual people in their own personal physical vehicles, who all have their own individual destinations.

Next, try to visualize a head-on view of a lot of motor vehicles in many lanes, all going up and down a couple of hills, then visualize an alternate view of a lot of people going up and down escalators (as, for example, in an airport or a large train station).

In the first instance, the drivers control the direction and speed of their vehicles, as well as their care, maintenance, and performance. Likewise, people are also the drivers of their own bodies, and they control the direction and speed of their journey, as well as the care, maintenance, and performance of their physical bodies.

Next, visualize three older vehicles next to one another. One is in excellent shape, one is worn out and broken down, and one has been wrecked in an accident. Then, visualize an alternate view of three older people. One is in excellent physical condition, one is worn out and slumped forward, and one is walking with crutches, wearing leg and arm casts and a neck brace.

The three motor vehicles have three basic destinies: to be well maintained and stay in good shape; to be poorly maintained and gradually break down, becoming increasingly unusable; or to be damaged in a sudden motor vehicle collision.

In the same way, our bodies also have several basic destinies: to be well cared for and maintained with appropriate habits, biomechanics, nutrition, rest, exercise, and so on; to become gradually broken down due to poor habits and maintenance; or to be injured suddenly.

Trucks and other motor vehicles can be repaired and the body can heal, but whether it involves a motor vehicle or the human body, the choice in all these cases is the driver's.

COMPARING TRUCK BODIES TO HUMAN BODIES

Essentially, humans created levers, wheels, wedges, and machines as extensions of themselves so they could improve their abilities and performance. From tennis shoes, to trucks, to spaceships, we have used our innovative talents to advance ourselves and society, and experience more of our surroundings.

Much of what we invented as extensions of ourselves has been patterned after our own bodies. For example, fulcrums, hinges, levers, and pulleys can be found in one form or another in our arms, elbows, shoulders, and tendons. Combinations of these devices we created form more complex inventions, such as computers, engines, and turbines, all with the purpose of facilitating human life.

Trucks, for example, enable us to travel farther, faster, and with much more stuff than we could possibly carry by ourselves. The truck is a synergistic combination of systems patterned, in many ways, after the human body. Interestingly, we get so caught up in the world around us that we have lost sight of how our own bodies (which are much more valuable than any truck) truly need to be taken care of. Consequently, we often see humans with poorly maintained, broken-down bodies, driving well-cared-for, high-performance vehicles.

It is now time to learn from our own inventions, the motor vehicles that enable us to move about better and faster. We need to apply the simple, yet powerful, techniques for vehicle care and maintenance to our own body vehicles that physically transport us along our roads in life. This is the crux of our book and we have based it on the BioErgonomic Safety Theory.

THE BEST WAY TO LEARN

The BioErgonomic Safety Theory (B.E.S.T.) was developed over time and has been implemented at the Carnegie Mellon Driver Training and Safety

Institute (CM-DTSI). The mission of CM-DTSI was to research and develop sustainable transportation safety that is both practical and economically feasible, through accident avoidance and prevention. This applies to both the prevention of motor vehicle accidents and the prevention of accidents to the physical body. Accidents occur as a series of events that, for our discussions, produce injury or other damage. Accidents, such as a slip, a fall, or a lifting strain, can occur precipitously, but they can also occur gradually with the repetition of poor habits, postures, or body movements.

The guiding premise of this bioergonomic systematic approach is preventive. Its aim is to help you achieve a personal sense of wellness and a state of comfortable safety by perfecting your understanding of, and the skills involved in, your body's movement in order to achieve a personal synergy and ultimately improve your quality of life.

In order to benefit most from this approach, you must thoroughly comprehend what your current level of understanding and use of your body is and how it interacts with the surrounding environment. Only then will you be able to take full advantage of this book and learn, from the many techniques and concepts it lays out for you, how to dramatically improve your knowledge, habits, and health.

ERGONOMICS

In any discussion of the BioErgonomic Safety Theory (B.E.S.T.), we must begin by defining ergonomics. Basically, it is the science of how to make your environment and body fit together well.

To most people, the word "ergonomic" means the ergonomically designed contour of a seat designed specifically to provide the most beneficial fit for a person's body. But, in fact, the visible seat is the last element of all the ergonomic industrial processes designed to produce a less stressing activity, whether this activity is connected to work, relaxation, or sleep.

Any activity of the body, including thinking, eating, moving, or even resting, has a cost in terms of energy. In our very first second of life outside the womb, we breathe oxygen, and throughout our entire lives, we constantly inhale, process, and exhale in order to live. In the course of this, we are consuming energy. The heart is consuming energy by pumping to circulate fresh oxygenated blood to all our other vital organs that, in turn, consume it to function as they are designed to.

The unit of measure that is applied to all the body's efforts is called the *erg*. One erg is the quantity of energy needed to elevate one gram of water by one calorie. An ergonomist is a person who observes and measures all the components of the simultaneous actions and interactions of the human body, for example, breathing, thinking, and running at the same time.

Ergonomics is a scientific discipline studying men and women in their occupational activities. It is a technology that takes its knowledge from everywhere, and it becomes an art when it applies this knowledge in order to transform an existing reality into a concept for the future, mainly in the field of protecting the health and safety of workers in the workspace.

The physical, mental, psychological, and social well-being of the workers must also be taken into account in order to help each person develop in their professional capacity during their active and productive life.

The word "ergonomic" was first used in 1857 by W. Jastrzebowski, a Polish man who published *Ergonomics: Draft of a Science for Working Conditions*. He describes ergonomics as the science of the use of strength and human capacity, and one hundred years later, an English engineer named K.F.H. Murrel defined the concept more precisely by getting recognition for this scientific multidiscipline and creating The Ergonomic Research Society, which was equally composed of physiologists, psychologists, and engineers (today, ergonomics is at the intersection of all these disciplines, along with biotechnology and socioeconomics).

Although ergonomics has expanded in many industrialized countries since then, there has not, so far, been a clear definition of the most important parameters for safety conditions during occupational activities.

B.E.S.T

The BioErgonomic Safety Theory combines the biological and the psychophysiological elements of ergonomics. The science of biology deals with living plants and animals, and the way they live and grow.

Every person has a biological signature, a personal way to react to their workload and its physical and psychological demands. Each person's biological needs are constant and cannot be changed without incurring risks. In order to perform at their best under optimal conditions, every person's physical and mental capacity should also be in a comfort zone for them. Similarly, for a car, if the engine runs too low or too high, there will soon be bad results, with possible stress and malfunctions. The comfort zone is the most efficient operating condition for the person and takes the least effort to operate more smoothly and therefore longer.

B.E.S.T., the BioErgonomic Safety Theory, combines the biological and ergonomic components of the person (that is, physiological, psychological, sociological) in order to develop a more energy-saving model to optimize the person's resources and produce the maximum impact on work at the minimum effort level, within a person's comfort zone. This also describes the most efficient and energy-conserving routine for a person to perform their given tasks at an optimal sustainable level. For example, at CM-DTSI, a popular driving course is on economical driving (how to save gas). One of the aims of our book is to try and do the same thing for people. We want to help people use their bodies most efficiently so they can conserve their energy and therefore have more of it for other tasks, with less wear and tear on their bodies, and enough energy in reserve for any unexpected event that requires more energy.

B.E.S.T. takes the demands of the job into consideration, as well as the person's capabilities in real-life conditions before and after work. The ability to rest, relax, rejuvenate, and recuperate after work is a very important element that cannot be altered without danger. B.E.S.T. has developed methods to evaluate and train each person to appreciate his or her level of comfort, and to understand the level of danger if and when the optimum conditions for operating the body are not maintained.

This BioErgonomic Safety Theory emphasizes ergonomical human performances and the limits in real daily-life situations and activities. As the environment changes so, too, do the person's input/output capabilities.

Thanks to the technological progress of computerized contemporary life, we can now simultaneously measure a lot of parameters with precise, infinite, minute details. Now, more than ever, we can describe the interconnections between our minds and our bodies.

Today, stress, fatigue, and alertness can be measured. The level of noises, vibrations, heat, and complex visual multitasking can be recorded and instantly correlated with other data monitoring: heartbeats, blood pressure, breathing, sweating, and the variation of internal temperature in order to evaluate the efforts performed by those on the job, always being vigilant about safety.

GETTING AROUND

How we get around in the world relates not only to our mode of transportation, but also to our bodies and their mechanical efficiency. Even realizing that the human body is much more complex and miraculous than a truck, we can use the analogy of truck versus body because it is how we use and care for each that determines the quality of life and longevity of each.

What it takes to keep a truck viable over an extended period of time is much the same, in principle, as keeping your body moving and thriving. Like a truck, how you manage your body, how you take care of it, and how well you know it will determine how well and how long you survive.

How many miles do you have left?

SCRAP METAL OR COLLECTOR'S ITEM?

The passing of time is not the only thing that makes us age. Just as a truck will fail when it is neglected and abused, so we will age faster when our bodies are not functioning at their best, when we are malnourished, and when we neglect signs of ill health.

If you misuse a truck, it gets rusty and broken down before long, and winds up being towed to a scrap heap. If you misuse a body, it gets wrinkled and stiff-jointed, and winds up going to an early grave. If, on the other hand, you take care of a truck, follow regular maintenance routines, keep it clean and well-oiled, it can last for decades and decades, eventually becoming a collectible antique. The same holds for your body. If you take care of it, follow regular maintenance routines, and keep it clean and well-oiled, it could easily last a century or more. According to the American Academy of Sciences, our bodies are designed to last 125 years. That, however, takes a little effort, although there are now 70,000 people in the United States who are 100 or over, and recent figures indicate that centenarians are the fastest growing demographic group.

RESTORATION *IS* POSSIBLE

Some people say, "It's too late. The damage is done." On the contrary, with the right attitude and good effort, it is not too late to change the way you use your body. It's not too late to correct bad posture, bad diet, and other bad habits that are literally sucking the life out of you. Just as it is possible to restore an old truck and bring it back to the magnificence of its youth, it is also possible to restore the efficiency and health of your body.

As we explore the basic components of keeping and maintaining good health, we will look closely at balance, form, flow, time, repetition, force, and flexibility. These seven topics are fundamental to any understanding of good health and good truck maintenance.

MIND AND BODY IN TRUCKS AND DRIVERS

We also need to consider for a moment the correlation between the truck and the driver. For all practical purposes, the mind of the truck is the driver. Although a truck performs many automatic, programmed functions, it cannot think for itself, but with the aid of computerized monitoring systems, the truck can communicate with the driver through a series of gauges and indicator lights. Still, when it comes to the operation and maintenance decisions, those can only be made by the driver and the mechanic.

As the mind of the truck, the driver responds to roads, traffic, location, weather conditions, day versus night driving, and whether or not there is a full load when determining how to handle the truck. If the truck overheats, the driver gives it a rest and tends to its maintenance. If the truck needs fuel or oil, the driver sees to it. If the truck shows signs of stress or engine trouble, the driver takes steps to remedy the situation.

How well a driver knows the vehicle and its communication devices and, given that awareness, how well he treats it determines in large part the fitness and well-being of the truck.

Your body also has a driver: your mind. Though you do not come with gauges and indicator lights, you do have the ability to recognize what your body needs, and it does communicate with you. When you are tired, you should recognize that fact and rest. When you are hungry, you should recognize that fact and eat. When you are sore, stiff, in pain, or have other symptoms, you should be aware of them, acknowledge them, and respond to your needs.

The next time you climb into a truck or any vehicle, take a minute to look at what is now a sophisticated piece of machinery. It is an elaborate combination of mechanical and electronic technology. Think about how it compares to your body and mind, which are also sophisticated combinations of mechanical and neurological systems that must work in harmony in order to sustain your quality of life and your longevity.

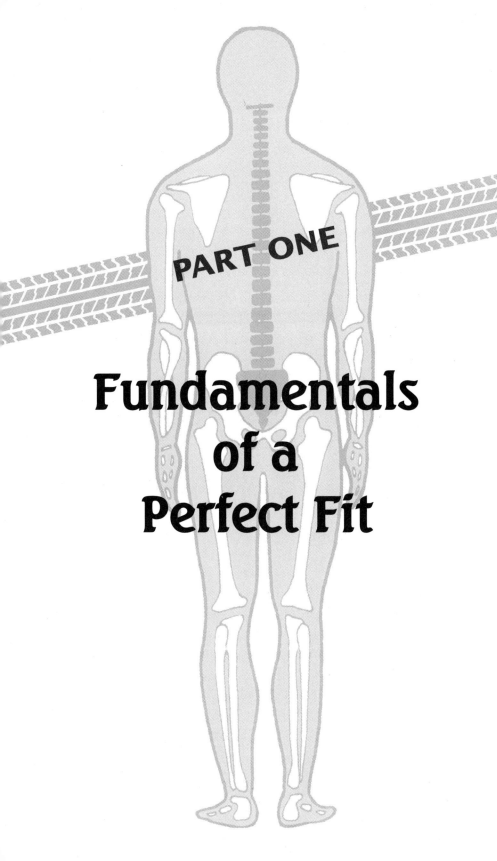

PART ONE

Fundamentals of a Perfect Fit

1. AGING

Of all the health problems facing society today, aging—especially premature aging of the physical body and its many related conditions—is the principal one that will confront each of us sooner or later.

The common, staggering statistic that 80 percent of Americans will suffer debilitating back pain at some point in their lives does not indicate a design flaw in the body, but rather a flaw in our understanding and use of our bodies. Premature physical aging, like recurring back pain, is largely preventable.

As early as 1983, the American Academy of Sciences said the human body should be able to last at least a healthy 125 years. If we do not directly address key processes that decrease our ability, cause pain, and accelerate structural aging, the experience of living more years—in comfort, in health, and with dignity—will not be attainable.

I have been in active practice for more than seventeen years, and have seen people's bodies decline in the different phases of life, yet I have also witnessed many people heading down that path who are able to reverse and seemingly defy the aging process.

We all understand how orthodontic braces apply pressure and force to redirect the growth pattern of teeth and improve their function and aesthetic appeal. Conversely, if braces were applied to properly aligned, well-functioning teeth, these straight teeth could be made to grow crooked over time.

On the other end of the body, we all understand that athletic shoes must be precisely fit to the individual wearer's unique foot size and arch contours, as well as to the type of activity for which the shoes are intended.

The wrong size and type of shoe would certainly impair athletic performance and foot health.

Why are these seemingly simple concepts so easy to understand about teeth and feet, but not about the rest of the body in between?

GETTING OFF ON THE WRONG FOOT

With great anticipation, I pulled the edge-worn, yellow writing tablet from my briefcase on the first leg of a flight from Omaha to Raleigh, North Carolina, where I was speaking to a conference of business leaders. As I worked on my speech, I wanted to make my point about how our bodies conform to our environment—in many cases, to a poorly designed environment. But how?

I began to sketch the type of device needed to force an individual's right foot into the same type of environment that people's bodies are forced into over time. It wasn't difficult. I just had to look around the airplane. People of all sizes and shapes were shoehorned into same-sized seats. The answer was obvious. I made new notes for my speech.

I eagerly began my presentation at this lively, well-attended conference by asking the participants to take off their shoes. As we all took them off, there was an instantaneous mingling of people wondering what was next. I asked everyone to hold their right shoe in their right hand and place it on their left foot. I then asked them to put their left shoes on their right feet and stand up.

As we all stood, most people were leaning forward looking at their shoes and commenting on how awkward and unusual they felt.

I then asked: *What if you grew up wearing shoes like this?* (See Figure 1.1.) What if you thought it was normal because everybody else did it? By the time you got to your present age, wouldn't your feet have grown abnormally? Wouldn't you have had more problems, perhaps begun to develop

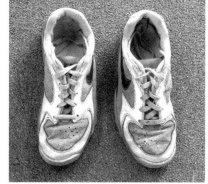

Figure 1.1. What would your feet look like if you always wore your shoes on the opposite feet?

arthritis? Wouldn't your walking and running be impaired? And wouldn't the pain interfere with your rest or relaxation?

This is precisely what was been happening to our bodies—in particular, to our backs—throughout the course of our lives. We've been trying to wear our bodies on the wrong foot:

➤ At poorly fitting workstations;

➤ In the wrong-sized chairs;

➤ In car seats that are too small or too big;

➤ In uncomfortable restaurant booths and awkward patio furniture;

➤ In front of computer screens, especially laptops, that are at the wrong level;

➤ In hotel beds that are too soft or too hard;

➤ In airline seats where one size fits "a few";

➤ Standing in line, leaning over a grocery cart;

➤ Reaching for telephones that are too far away;

➤ Gardening, sweeping, washing the car, and vacuuming;

➤ Reading in bed and watching a TV that's improperly positioned;

➤ Improperly lifting, and paying the price with back pain later;

➤ Carrying all kinds of items improperly, including purses, luggage, backpacks, and briefcases;

➤ Purchasing and wearing clothing that continues to put our bodies into the "wrong shoe."

I made my point with the business leaders in North Carolina, and I hope to make my point in this book. There is good news—although this process of postural and physical decline is common, it is not necessary. I firmly believe the human body was intended to age in a graceful and healthy manner. The aging process was not designed to inflict pain and regret on the process of life. We've begun to reengineer our workplaces. Now, let's reengineer our own environment and the way we interact with it so we will improve our destiny.

AGING WELL

How long do you want to live? The common answer is, "As long as I have a sharp mind and a healthy body." If we're lucky, we watch our grandparents and parents age gracefully. However, sometimes it's not so graceful. Sometimes they battle chronic conditions that restrict their ability to walk, move around their own homes, or dress themselves. We witness daily activities becoming difficult, if not impossible, for many of our senior citizens.

You might turn to your children and say, "Don't let me get like that." But whose responsibility is it to keep your body in the best possible shape to last your lifetime? It's your responsibility, of course. And, believe it or not, you do have a certain measure of control over how well you age.

HOW TO AGE WELL

If we expect to live as long as we are designed to, and live as healthy and satisfying a life as possible—particularly the second half—then we need to modify many of our actions and habits right now. It's never too late.

The body's natural tendency is toward health and it will naturally search out the best conditions for health and longevity when given the awareness and the proper opportunity to do so. You have to provide the right mindset to promote health, and then be sure to include a high enough intake of oxygen to ensure that all the body's tissues become, and stay, refreshed. Next, it's up to you to take in the appropriate quantities and varieties of nutrients to be the building blocks of the physical body. It's also your job to make sure they are digested properly so they can reach the areas where they are needed.

THE DIFFERENCE BETWEEN A GOOD FIT AND A POOR FIT

If it is appropriate to do so, take off both your shoes. Switch them, putting your right shoe on your left foot and your left shoe on your right foot. If they are lace-up shoes, retie them. Just be careful not to use high heels with this exercise.

Now stand up and press down slightly, first on your left foot, then on your right. Concentrate fully on how your feet feel inside your reversed shoes. Carefully roll up on your toes and back on your heels. Hold on to something for balance if necessary. Sit down again and concentrate fully on your feet. Feel how the shoe rubs and pushes against your large toe and the front part of your inside arch. Feel also how your heel is probably turned inward. Notice how the outside of your foot is being pushed inward by the arch support and how your toes tend to point outward. Roll your ankles inward and notice how your arch would flatten if allowed to remain inside your opposite shoes.

If you keep your feet in these reversed shoes long enough, you will also notice how the lower leg twists slightly and causes your knees to turn and rotate inward. If you walk for any length of time like this, you will notice cramping across the bottom of the arch, possibly in the calf, and there will be strain in your ankles.

Imagine if you had worn your shoes like this from the day you began wearing shoes. Your feet would actually conform to the contour of the shoes you wore every day, all day. Picture yourself trying to run and play on the playground, jumping up and down, and performing sporting activities with your feet supported this way.

DEFORM TO CONFORM

With the shoes switched like this, your feet would eventually deform to conform since they were not being supported in their natural form. Degenerative changes would be inevitable. Circulation in your feet would be altered, and your ability to play sports or just walk, stand, and do just about every other activity would be adversely affected. Ultimately, if you lived long enough, you would hardly be able to walk.

If everyone wore their shoes reversed, then there would be degeneration, poor performance, and other foot problems in everybody's life. Most people conditioned to these problems from a early age would experience the problems of pain and poor health, and would, amazingly, accept the pain rather than question it and start to undo the current damage and prevent further damage. Your feet might have looked quite deformed had this process happened to you.

"How absurd," you say? "We would have never let this happen, we would have known better." But, ironically, this very phenomenon has already happened, not to our feet, but to the larger sections of our bodies.

TECHNOLOGY AND THE HUMAN CONDITION

The startling observation of how very poorly we used our bodies in the workplace became evident to me as early as 1982. I was working with patients who had difficulty fully recovering from their neck and back conditions until we began addressing their movement and their postural habits at work.

After observing many people in their workplaces, and noting that they overwhelmingly used postures and movements that directly aggravated their conditions, it became quite clear to me that people weren't understanding and using their bodies as they were designed to be used. In fact, once you understand how the body is designed to hold itself, move, work, and relax, you will probably find your current habits as absurd as the left shoe/right foot exercise, and wonder, how did we ever get this way in the first place?

It began with my observations at the workplace, but over time I also became aware of the implications and effects of poor postural habits and inattention to body positions during driving, sleeping, leisure, and at home activities. How we got this way in the first place goes as far back as the Industrial Revolution and its focus on mechanization and standardization in order to lower costs and mass-produce items. Left in its wake was a lack of understanding and respect for individual physical uniqueness and the fundamentals of good body mechanics.

What is the anthropological basis for poor postures? Were any civilizations successful at this? Unfortunately, prior to the Industrial Revolution, in the hunting and gathering days, or the Agricultural Revolution, our ancestors had a much shorter life expectancy, so the negative consequences of poor physical habits and inadequate healing from trauma did not matter because very few lived that long anyway. Today we are living to experience them and trying to do something about it.

Like fingerprints, no two human bodies are exactly the same in height, length, shape, or contour. Even similar body types may not be in similar physical condition, or have similar physical histories that would include fitness habits, heredity, or any injuries.

During our preoccupation with the Industrial Revolution, we gradually accumulated development problems from poor postures and biomechanically unsound movements in the workplace. Given that there was an overall lack of understanding of what proper rest, or aspects of proper physical care involved, and what their value was, we did not know to question what impact this would have on our bodies and our lives in the future. Further, the onset of problems was so gradual that mass standardization of them became culturally acceptable.

It has taken literally generations to understand the impact that lack of proper attention to our bodies and the way we interact with our environment has had on us, both as individuals and as a society. Our improper physical habits have become set by time and the repetition of the behaviors and actions of others learned during our formative years.

These habits contribute to the premature aging of the physical body, increased levels of stress and fatigue, and a lower quality of life. Couple this with the fact that we are living longer lives as a society and we quickly see what the quality of that increased life will be—not very good!

OUR BODIES' PHYSICAL NEEDS

Wrapped up in the process of day-to-day life as we are, through time we have simply lost touch with the physical needs of our bodies. We now seem to be paying the price for this unintentional neglect with pain, recurring physical injury, stress, fatigue, and probably avoidable degenerative changes. But there is a way to change things for the better.

The typical course of individual life, from the early years to the average life expectancy, is evident in how our bodies age (see Figure 1.2 on page 18). Physical habits that we acquire and perpetuate have a direct bearing on how our bodies matures and how, for most of us, it declines to the end of life. Your body can last a lifetime—your lifetime—and you can prepare now to physically navigate through your life to reach what many people think could be the life expectancy of our bodies, 120 years or more.

What physical requirements and habits will enable us to have a long and good life? Consider these goals as you read this section and you will be well on your way to helping yourself.

➤ Read so you can learn how to remove the unnecessary physical demands and strains on your body, and how to enjoy the benefits of taking such actions.

➤ Become aware of how you currently interact with your environment.

➤ Study the figures in this book, and watch how others fit or don't fit into their work, home, and leisure surroundings, and why.

THE BASIC FUNDAMENTALS

Although the concept of a perfect fit may seem impractical and unattainable, you can achieve a practically perfect fit by determining how your unique body and its needs can realistically fit into your current environment and physical surroundings in a way that makes your body healthier.

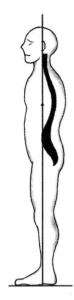 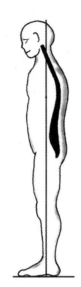 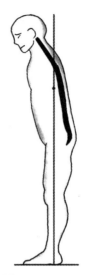 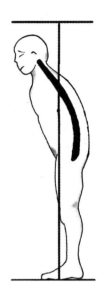

Figure 1.2

| From the side, the spine should have smooth flowing curves in an s-shaped pattern. | When the head moves forward of the gravity line, the curve in the neck flattens as does the curve in the lower back. | After the head has moved forward of the gravity line, gravity will gradually pull the head further forward, causing distortion of the upper and lower spine. | The end result of a lifetime of poor postural habits is often an increasingly slumping spine and body. |

To do this, we need to apply the basic fundamentals of physicality to most aspects of your daily life. They are:

- ➤ Balance
- ➤ Form
- ➤ Flow
- ➤ Time
- ➤ Repetition
- ➤ Force
- ➤ Flexibility

As you come to understand the effect of these fundamentals on your body and life, you will be in a perfect position to make the basically simple, yet profound and meaningful, changes needed to enhance your physical health and well-being.

2. BALANCE

Balance is defined as a state of equilibrium characterized by the cancellation of all forces by equal, opposing forces.

BALANCE AND ALIGNMENT IN TRUCKS AND HUMANS

How do you know if your truck is out of alignment? If the tires are out of balance? First, you might notice that the steering wheel pulls to one side, then you'll eventually notice uneven wear on the tires. These minor problems compound as time goes on and increase your risk of accidents when you encounter adverse road conditions or harsh weather. If the tires are disproportionately worn, with time their wear pattern will have an adverse impact on the axles and frame of the truck, creating extensive, costly damage to it. On the other hand, if you maintain the proper alignment and balance, your truck will handle more efficiently and you can maintain maximum control of it in unpredictable road and weather conditions.

Faulty alignment also affects the overall wear and tear on your truck. If it is pulling and bouncing to one side, that also puts unnecessary stress and strain on the axle and frame of your truck. And the longer the problem goes on, the more adverse its effect is on the performance of your truck.

Alignment is just as important for your body, and proper posture is the best way to keep your body in alignment. If, day after day, you lean against an armrest that is too low, too high, or too far away from your body, and you don't counteract that out-of-balance position with stretching or neutralizing movements, your body will eventually conform to that bent posture. Your muscles will conform to your distorted shape, and, with your alignment compromised, your body will stop functioning efficiently; if left unattended, it will eventually cause you pain.

If you are out of balance, there will be more wear and tear on your body as it adjusts itself to compensated movements, and it will be subject to decreased performance and movement, and further damage.

Let's compare worn shoes to worn tires. (See Figures 2.1 and 2.2.) Take a look at your favorite old shoes, the ones you like to slip into and spend time in. If they are unevenly worn on either the outside or the inside, they will affect your frame, and your ankles, knees, hips, and spine will have to compensate for the uneven platform you are standing on by shifting out of alignment to keep you balanced. In time, these compensating arrangements of your skeleton and muscles will compound themselves and become habitual. Even if you do put on a pair of well-fitting shoes, it will be too late at that point, and the end result will be poor performance in your connective tissues, internal organs, muscles, and, in fact, your entire body.

A poorly aligned body has an increased risk of injury during physical activity or movements involving quick reflexes, such as catching yourself if you trip or stumble. The longer your body is out of balance, the more you compromise your good health. You can learn to counteract the ill effects of poor alignment by practicing good posture, regular exercise, and stretching.

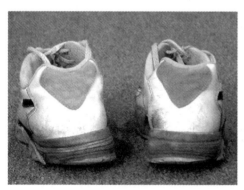

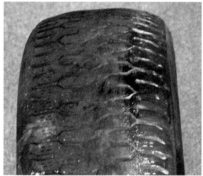

Figure 2.1. Uneven wear on shoes is a sign of imbalance.

Figure 2.2. Uneven wear on tires is a sign of imbalance or improper alignment.

BALANCE AND SHOCK ABSORPTION IN TRUCKS AND HUMANS

Trucks are designed with three elements for shock absorption: seats, suspension system, and tires. Seats are obviously for the comfort and posture of the driver; the suspension system and the tires are for the protection of the truck and all that it carries.

If a truck's suspension system is insufficient and the tires are under-inflated, the vehicle will bounce and shimmy its way down the road, making it more difficult to handle, especially if there is an unexpected obstacle on the road. Over time, a faulty suspension system can cause dispropor-tionate wear and tear on the truck and anything within it. The engine and frame would be rattled and the computerized monitoring systems would be compromised, not to mention the discomfort for the driver and any passengers.

Over long periods of time, vibrations have similarly negative effects on humans. Before air-ride suspensions were developed, many long-distance drivers had excessive kidney, neck, and back problems, but since their development, these instances have been greatly reduced.

Human bodies have many mechanisms for shock absorption. Muscles, tendons, ligaments, spinal discs, the s-shaped spinal curve, and the menis-cus cartilage in the knee can all work as air-ride suspension systems for the body. And, like trucks, these human shock absorbers all rely on proper bal-ance and alignment to function correctly. Leaning sideways or forward does not allow the spinal discs to absorb the impact of stepping, running, or bouncing.

When your personal shock absorbers are ineffective, damage is likely to occur in both your skeleton and your internal organs—the bladder, kid-neys, nervous system, prostate, or uterus for example. Like a truck, your frame is designed to hold your operating systems in their ideal position for maximum performance, and this proper alignment allows for efficient and effective shock absorption. When your frame is rattled around excessively, however, your systems can fail, but when those systems are working well, you will be alert and better able to focus on your job or any task you have to perform.

BALANCE ON A TEETER-TOTTER

Remember when you ran outside during recess in grade school, hopped up on one side of the teeter-totter, and one of your friends sat on the other end? It was a delicate balancing act, but when it worked, you would both be suspended in the air. Unless something happened to disturb that deli-cate balance, you could stay there throughout the entire recess. If one of you were to lean forward or backward and disrupt the balance, then the teeter-totter would tip in the other's favor. In order to achieve balance again, you would have to start over and work at it.

Balance in nature is relatively effortless when forces counteract each other equally. Imbalance is characterized by the need to expend energy to achieve balance again, or to maintain the imbalance. The phenomenon of physical balance in the human system is similar in many ways to the teeter-totter. Forces counteract each other to achieve balance and energy is thus conserved. Having a balanced state in the body can then become relatively effortless.

It is important to note that the best-balanced postures and positions must respect the design of the human body. For example, the spine is actually engineered to be able to achieve and maintain an upright, balanced posture relatively effortlessly when its own design is intact.

The spine is composed of twenty-four individual vertebrae that have a predetermined structural balance and alignment. Under normal conditions, the seven vertebrae in the neck (cervical spine) curve forward, as do the five vertebrae in the lower back (lumbar spine). These twelve vertebrae are counterbalanced by the twelve vertebrae in the mid-back (thoracic spine) moving backward. This is similar to stacking twelve bricks on the one side of a teeter-totter and twelve bricks on the other side.

When the spine is naturally aligned, then balance is achieved through the overall posture of the body. Viewed from the side, this natural alignment shows that the center of the hips follows a straight line through to the front part of the ankle. The shoulders move over the hips, and the head, or center of the ear, is positioned over the shoulders. Just for fun, check your own alignment in a full-length mirror.

FIRM FOUNDATION

The feet are the foundation and the body's first contact with the ground in achieving an upright position. Any imbalance in the feet, in terms of their rotating inward or outward, or having a poor position for proper arch support, will affect balance. The same concept of imbalance is true for hip, knee, and leg positions, as well as arm, hand, and shoulder movements.

It is one thing to know what good balance looks like, yet another to try to achieve it. It might not be as easy as it seems because most of us have long since developed the imbalanced conditions that brought us to this point. Throughout your life, your own habits and other forces may have been working against balance or posture, and conditioning your body to be out of balance.

A key point to remember is that your lower back's forward curve is determined by the tilt of your tailbone. Think of a properly tilted tailbone as a rocket-launching platform angled forward so the rocket launches through your midsection. If your tailbone is not tilted forward, it will cause the S-curve of your back to straighten when your body adjusts for balance. In that case, if your rocket were to launch, it would shoot straight up the trail of your vertebrae and hit you in the head in the form of headaches and back pain. That is a good reason to always remember to tilt your tailbone forward.

THE SECRET OF THE RIB CAGE

The secret to proper posture is in the forward and back rocking-chair-style rock of the rib cage. If your lower rib cage moves forward and your tailbone is tilted properly, then the upper ribcage moves backward in a better position. You create a nice forward curve in your lower back and your shoulders naturally fall back into place—without being forced.

Let's say you're told to stand up straight. What do you do? Frequently, people tighten their shoulders or pull their shoulder blades back together to achieve what they think is better posture. Try it. You'll find it feels forced and unnatural. As a way to achieve good posture, it is doomed to fail because you can't hold this position for long. If the rib cage is flattened or rocked in a position where the upper part of the rib cage is moved forward (in a slump), the shoulders cannot come back into a naturally balanced position.

Try this. Stand up and hook your thumbs behind your back so they touch the lower ribs (see Figure 2.3). Gently push forward on those lower ribs and allow the lower rib cage to rock forward and the upper ribs to rock backward.

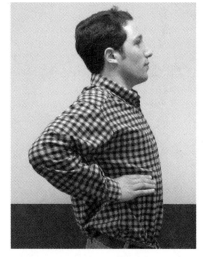

Figure 2.3. Place your thumbs at the level of the lower rib cage with your fingers pointing straight forward.

You will notice that your shoulders move back automatically over your hips because the shoulders are merely passengers on the rib cage.

You just did the Rib-Cage Rock. Notice that you raised your chin as your shoulders moved automatically over your hips. That is how good posture is supposed to feel.

This rib-cage position encourages greater lung capacity and allows more air to be inhaled deeper and more easily. This enhances oxygenation, which improves circulation of the blood to the rest of the body. Good shoulder and rib-cage position encourage your whole spine to assume its natural s-shaped curve. Balance and movement are easier in this position.

The head or neck posture (created by the forward curve of the cervical vertebrae) is best maintained with a level head. When you do this rib-cage position, note the positions of the chin and the ear in relation to the shoulders (see Figure 2.4). The chin should be level with the floor, with the head *not* extended so that the ear canal falls backward at the shoulder level. A level head allows good forward head posture and is a natural result of good positioning in the lower and mid-back. All too often, our head is tilted forward instead, as a result of our postural activities and our line of vision (see Figure 2.5). This posture causes the cervical spine to become flat or even reversed in its curve (see Figure 2.6).

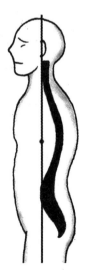
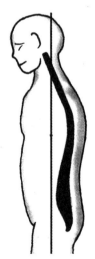
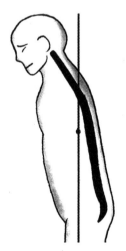

Figure 2.4. Note the positions of the chin and the ear in relation to the shoulders.

Figure 2.5. Note forward tilt of the head as a result of postural activities and line of vision.

Figure 2.6. Forward tilt of the head causes the cervical spine to become flat or even reversed in its curve.

MAXIMIZING RIB-CAGE AND CORE-BODY STRETCHES

Here is an excellent way to maximize the effectiveness of stretching in the key areas around the lower rib cage to improve posture and body mechanics, and also improve the health of the lower back. Follow the steps below closely. Consult your doctor if you have any questions before starting these exercises.

Side Body Stretches

1. Place your left hand at the level of your waist with your palm down (see Figure 2.7).

2. Push your hip to the right with your left hand until you feel a stretch on your right side, then stop. Now put your right arm straight up over your head and stretch with your right arm until you feel a pulling along the entire right side (see Figure 2.8).

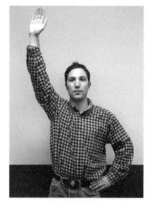

Figure 2.7

3. Breathe in deeply then exhale slowly to gain additional stretching on the right side, and make sure your head is tilted to the left along with your entire upper body. Come back toward the center and repeat the stretch again five times. Be sure to hold each part of the stretch for a short time before you go on to the next step, and make sure you continue to feel the stretch spread along your hip and side with each subsequent stretch.

4. With your right hand on your right hip, taking deep breaths at the appropriate time, slowly repeat this exercise five times for the left side.

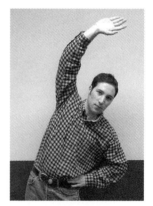

Figure 2.8

Side Rib-Cage Stretch

1. Now put your left hand, palm down, at the level of the lower rib cage, about six inches up from where you had your hand placed on your hip (see Figure 2.9).

2. Push your rib cage to the right with your left hand until you feel the

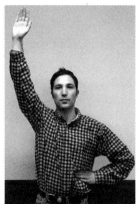

Figure 2.9

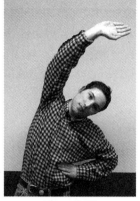

Figure 2.10

stretch across your right rib cage and side. Then, still pushing the rib cage with the left hand, bring your right arm over your head and stretch toward the left, tilting your head to the left at the same time (see Figure 2.10). Hold that position until you feel the stretch move up higher on your rib cage and side.

3. Now take a deep breath, hold it for a few seconds, and exhale. Repeat this stretch five times.

4. Put your right hand on the right side of your lower rib cage, about six inches up from where you had it placed on your right hip, and repeat the stretching pattern five times for the other side.

Back Extension

Combining the side-body and rib-cage stretch with the back and rib-cage extension exercises will enhance your efforts to improve your posture.

1. Placing the palms of your hands at the level of your waist on your lower back (see Figure 2.11), carefully push your hips forward until you feel a slight stretching in your lower back.

2. Move your upper back backward until you feel slightly more stretch in the lower back, and

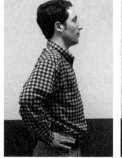

Figure 2.11

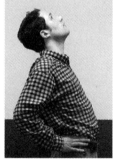

Figure 2.12

do not bend your knees (see Figure 2.12). Do not extend until you feel pain, only until you feel the stretch.

3. Now breathe in slowly and deeply, holding this breath for a few seconds, then breathe out and come to a upright position.

4. Repeat this stretch five times, breathing slowly and deeply throughout each stretch.

Lower Rib-Cage Extension Stretch

1. Now move your hands up about six inches from where they were placed in the lower back extension stretch and hook your thumbs around your lower rib cage (see Figure 2.13).

2. Move your rib cage forward by pushing with your thumbs against your rib cage until you feel a stretch at the lower rib cage.

3. Push your shoulders and head slightly backward to increase the extension of your lower rib cage (see Figure 2.14).

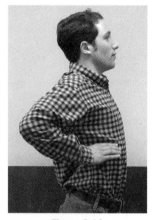

Figure 2.13

4. When you feel a good stretch, hold the position, then breathe in deeply, exhale slowly, and come back to the upright position. Repeat that stretch five times.

Back extension and lower rib-cage lateral stretching and extension are among the most overlooked stretches and movements in our daily activities. These stretches can be done in a very short period of time and should ideally be performed two to four times a day. As with any stretching and exercise program, if you experience pain, dizziness, weakness, or any discom-

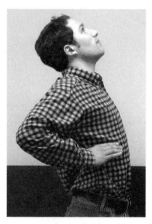

Figure 2.14

fort, discontinue immediately. If you have any health problems, or any questions about these activities, consult your healthcare provider before starting any stretching or exercise program.

MAINTAIN BALANCE

What sabotages your ability to maintain your best body position? Here are a few candidates.

1. **Line of Sight.** Your computer monitor is not directly in front of you, or the TV is on the dresser to the side of your bed. Your neck has to accommodate—sometimes with pain—to your sideways view.

2. **Visual Acuity.** It's amazing what a proper eye exam can uncover and correct. You may not even know how much difficulty you have seeing near or far until you have your sight corrected with contacts or glasses. Your posture can be drastically and adversely affected by leaning forward or backward to see something, like a computer screen, more clearly. This is a potential problem that is preventable.

3. **Reach of Arms and Legs.** The new car is great, but if the armrests don't fit naturally, you are forced to slump to the right when you drive so you can rest your arm on the console. A few simple adjustments of the seat (and that may mean using a pillow or rolled towel) may improve your posture and also make it easier for your feet to reach the pedals. (See Chapter 12 on driving for more information.)

4. **Asymmetrical Physical Structure.** Genetically, you may have one leg shorter than the other, or you may be living with the discomfort and imbalance of a broken leg from childhood that stunted the growth of that bone.

5. **Asymmetrical Physical Movements.** Golf is refreshing and relaxing, but it does focus movements on one side of your body more than the other. And reaching for the phone on one side of your desk—time after time, day after day—will also put you off balance.

6. **Deforming to Conform to the Environment.** Trying to make your body fit those stylish office chairs or high-fashion shoes is a formula for pain. So too are repetitive movements, such as lifting a child to your hip or shoulders, or carrying briefcases, lopsided book bags, or laptops every day.

7. **Preconditioned Habits.** It's the way you curl up on the couch, or in your favorite chair, or on the floor. These customary, yet improper, positions can cause imbalance, and if they are habits you get into a lot, they could affect you a lot by becoming chronic physical problems.

I often lecture to professionals about posture, and one day a colleague asked this thought-provoking question: "If I spend half my time slumping forward and half my time slumping backward, would they cancel each other out? And would I then be balanced?" "Not so," I responded. "If you look at the lumbar spine during forward and backward slumping, you'll note the lower back hasn't changed, it is flattened the same way in each position, so they would *compound* each other, not cancel each other out."

THE EFFECT OF DAILY LIVING

Sit forward in the chair you are in right now. Tilt your tailbone forward so your lower back curves forward. Put the back of your left hand in the hollow area of your lower back and then tilt your head forward. If you concentrate on where the back of your hand touches the muscles of your back and you tilt your head forward, you will notice there is muscle activity.

Arms and legs represent strong, effective levers. They may change position with respect to your sitting, standing, walking, and your related activities and actions at home, at leisure, during work, and with transportation. The core of the body, from the hips to the head, should be able to hold a position of balance throughout the course of your day's activities, but often doesn't.

If you examine what happens to your body during a typical day, you will be able to gain a better perspective on time's influence in eroding your physical health and well-being.

TIP THE SCALE IN YOUR FAVOR

Another aspect to balance in the human body: When forces counteract other forces to hold a position, they must be done in line with the way the body was engineered or designed. You could, for instance, achieve a balanced position by slumping forward, if the amount of backward movement in the low back and lower part of your rib cage counterbalanced the forward position of the upper rib cage and your head. This position would, however, not be in sync with the design of the body (see Figure 2.15).

This concept of balance also includes the optimum contact that the bones of the human frame have with one another for a given posture or movement. When the bones of the spine are balanced correctly, they have an optimum surface contact with one another that gives them the maximum

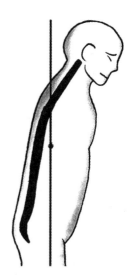

Figure 2.15. Trying to achieve a balanced position by slumping forward is not in sync with the body's design.

strength and safety for any given activity, such as lifting, sitting, or sleeping. Properly balanced, the bones of the wrist likewise have an optimum position to contact one another for best movement and maximum efficiency, with the least amount of friction. Every activity—from typing, fishing off a boat, sitting in a car or stadium seat, to mowing a lawn, using a computer mouse, or picking up a baby—has an optimum range of posture and movement that is safe and practical. (Study the following illustrations to understand this basic concept, and then apply them to your activities.)

Returning to the analogy of the teeter-totter in the playground, it functions best when its plank is perpendicular to the fulcrum underneath the plank. The teeter-totter would not be able to move and function well if its balance wasn't in accordance with the way it was designed to function.

If you were astride a teeter-totter where the plank was set at a thirty-degree angle to the support beam, you would have an awkward time trying to go up and down. Plus, the teeter-totter probably would not last long because stresses would develop in the plank that would cause it to break or splinter over time.

With respect to balance, the positions of your arms and legs have meaning not only in terms of the leverage they provide (see Figure 2.16), but also in terms of the balance points they have within their ranges of motion. The range of motion of the shoulder, for instance, has a balance point at which it functions best, depending upon what task it is performing. And the same is true for the forearms, the wrists, the knees, the hips, and the feet.

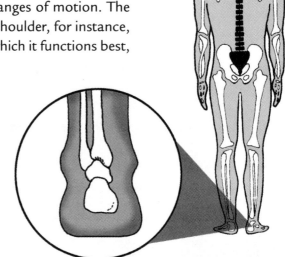

Figure 2.16. There is a normal balance between the left and right sides of the body so that weights and pressures can be evenly distributed along the hips, legs, and feet.

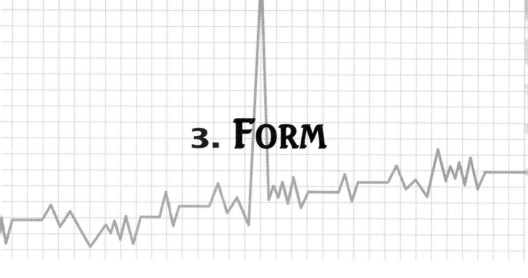

3. FORM

F orm can be defined as the shape and structure of something, as distinguished from its substance; the essence of something, as distinguished from its matter.

FORM AND FUNCTION IN TRUCKS AND HUMANS

Trucks come in a variety of sizes and shapes, each designed for specific tasks, or to haul different types of cargo. There are small trucks for short distance deliveries, and medium-sized trucks, such as vans, refrigerator, and dry-box trucks. Then there are the mammoth flatbed trucks, which are generally customized for specific tasks and different conditions and locations. Some are designed to be wind resistant, some are designed for flat country, and some for mountainous terrain. There are trucks for hauling lightweight or hazardous materials; and some of the largest are used to transport heavy machinery and construction materials.

When choosing which type of truck to use for a specific load, the first consideration is the weight and size of the load. In other words, what kind of task is involved? Your second consideration would be the distance and terrain to be covered. You wouldn't use a shortbed truck to carry twenty tons of I-beams from Detroit across the plains and two mountain ranges to Los Angeles. If you tried, you would most likely wind up with blown tires, engine failure, and large fines, and you could possibly cause a serious accident.

Proper truck selection is paramount in preventing accidents and successfully completing any task.

Look around you, it should come as no surprise that we humans come in an assortment of sizes and shapes. Although we are not designed to be "task specific," we must consider what types of tasks we might be best suited for, and how well we would function under different circumstances. For instance, for many people, staying awake and alert when driving long distances could be a problem, so these people would not want to consider long-haul trucking.

When considering a particular task, we need to take our physical shape and condition, as well as our mental abilities, into account. Though much of our physical shape is inherited, how it develops as we go through life is very much a product of our lifestyle and habits. Unlike a truck with one specific purpose, we can change our bodies to better prepare them for a variety of specific tasks. We can increase our stamina, we can properly align our bodies, and we can condition our muscles for lifting and sitting erect.

Proper conditioning of the body is essential for the prevention of injury and chronic illness. Proper lifting techniques, regular exercise, appropriate diet, and relaxation allow us to maintain and promote good form and function in our given bodies.

THE SHAPE YOU'RE IN

In the flow of life, we have a form. It comes first and the other fundamentals act on it, so if you understand how to manipulate the principles that influence form, you can change the form.

The visible form of your physical body is unique in its size, shape, and contour. Also inherent in the word "form" is the shape and condition of your body which is actually a combination of your heredity and your habits.

Take a moment and stand in front of a large mirror. Look at your true visible form. Do this nude, in a swimsuit, or in clothes that allow you to see not the body you want it to be, or the one you believe it will be, but your true body. For now, look at its form just for what it is. Don't be critical. This is the form you must fit into your environment. The more you know your own form, the better you will be able to make it fit into your life and your environment.

➤ Look straight ahead, into the mirror. Observe the posture of your head. Is it tilted to the side or rotated?

➤ Look down your neck and across your shoulders. Are they the same height? Is one higher and narrower than the other?

➤ Relax your arms by your side and look to see if there is an increase in space between the inside of your arms and the sides of your body. Is there a difference in space from one side to the other? Do your arms hang evenly?

➤ Look at the shape of your chest, your sides, rib cage, and abdomen and notice how that all changes as you get to your hips and upper thighs.

➤ Observe the contour of your thighs and knees. Note if they are the same size, or in the same position on each side.

➤ Look at the contour and shape of your knees, your thighs, and your feet. What is the shape and contour of your feet, and do they match each other? Are your ankles turned inward, your feet pointed out, your knees knocked inward, or your hips turned on one side more than the other?

Take a thorough look at the form of your body and get a good understanding of the shape. Now turn sideways and, as best as you can, look at the form of the front of your body, from your head, across your body, past your legs, to your feet. Now check the back part of your neck, shoulders, and mid-back. Move your eyes down through your lower back, hips, and legs.

Your form has been hardened or weakened by a lifetime of habits, which include activities, inactivity, injuries, movements, postures, and the strains and stresses that have accumulated throughout the course of a lifetime. Your weakened form may not be life-threatening, but it is certainly lifestyle threatening.

To a large extent, habits have formed you. But you can change your form with conscientious effort and a clear understanding of how to fit your form into your surroundings and how to modify your surroundings to better fit your form.

I will discuss how to harness the power of time and repetition to assist you. For now, learn to know the nature of your form and compare what you have learned with the progression of physical decline that occurs with aging (see Figure 1.2 on page 18). When you do this, you will have an idea in what direction you are heading.

CHANGE YOUR MIND FIRST

Up to this time, your form has been unintentionally shaped to be the way it is. The exciting news is that you can change your form, your physical destiny, by first becoming aware of and then changing your actions and adopting different, beneficial types of activities, movements, and postures.

Once you become aware how important it is to make needed changes, you can then start making them in your routine and your environment. With this book, you are starting what some researchers call "precontemplation." The information here will help you move from contemplation, to preparation, to action. These are logical and normal stages of change, and they're easy *once you get started*. In essence, you actually set yourself up to change.

In many cases, it requires changing your mind to make your habits and actions change (the cognitive approach). For some, however, it is very difficult to change their minds or change their habits. In those cases, changing actions first (in a behavioral manner) and then feeling how those changes affect both form and comfort can lead to improvements because the results demonstrate that these actions are helpful in the short-term and long-term, and that then changes your mind.

Whether you change your mind or change your actions first, depending on whichever is easier for you, either will lead you to the same result. Keep in mind that when you're making changes to better support your form in your home. workplace, and transportation, you must consider not only what fits for your current condition, but also what will be necessary to improve your form.

A WORD ABOUT WELL-BEING

We use the word "well-being" and the phrase "health and well-being" to mean the physical, mental, and emotional state in which you are best able to express yourself and your unique talents and abilities in order to accomplish your personal goals.

Premature structural aging limits both the quantity and quality of life. It distracts your attention, and takes time and energy away from accomplishing your goals. It takes the fun, and often much of the meaning, out of life.

If certain areas of your body have become tight because of habits, movements, and postures, it is important to make changes, not just in your environmental support, but also in your exercising, stretching, and relaxation regimens. Most of us have developed habits or actions that require our bodies to be slumped forward in space more often and more repetitively than they are extended backward in space. For example, such common actions as bending over to tend to children, tie shoes, drive a car, or read a book that is on your lap or on a desk all involve slumping forward.

The predominant changes needed to restore balance to your form include improving the inward curve of the lower back, the positioning of the rib cage, and the positioning of the head and neck. Because most of the things we do require forward movements, compensating extension activities must be incorporated into your daily life. These could include adopting open sleeping postures (see Figure 3.1) with extension stretches beforehand, leaning back in a swing, or standing in a doorway, holding your arms out parallel to the floor and letting them press against the door frame.

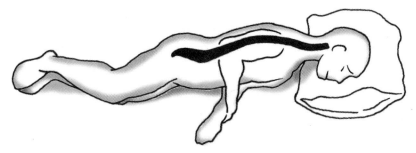

Figure 3.1. An open sleeping posture allows the natural flow of spinal curves to remain intact during sleep.

Although individual circumstances always exist and there are exceptions to every rule, the overwhelming trend in physical body movement, postures, and habits is similar for most of us and is described throughout this book. Your situation may well require working with your healthcare professional to accomplish your goals.

If inactivity, stress, and continual adoption of forward postures have hardened your form, it will take time for it to readjust to its natural and rightful position. Basically, you never reach a point when you can cease your activities because your actions, movements, and habits are either carrying you toward poor health or toward better health and well-being. You have an opportunity now to take a look at exactly what has been happening to you unconsciously, without even thinking, and be able to make conscious changes to actually move your physical health in the direction you want it to go.

4. FLOW

The technical definition of flow is to move with a continual shifting of the component particles. But in a larger sense, flow is life, and when flow is disturbed, then life is disturbed.

FLOW AND CIRCULATION IN TRUCKS AND HUMANS

Airflow and compression are key ingredients for efficient performance in a truck's engine. Decreased airflow adversely affects fuel consumption and the combustion process. More important, insufficient air supply causes a dangerous buildup of carbon dioxide and carbon monoxide levels in the exhaust system that can make their way to the vehicle's driver. To ward off any critical problems with air supply, it is important to maintain clean air filters and air intake systems.

Other components of a truck—air brakes, air horns, and the air conditioner—also depend on air, each of which contributes to the well-being of the driver and the safety of the truck and its cargo.

For humans, air is the single most important thing needed to sustain life. You can survive weeks without food, days without water, but deprive yourself of air for a very few minutes and death is imminent. Lungs are like air filters; they clean the bad stuff out with each breath we take. The air moves from our lungs to our heart, through our bodies, back to the heart, then through the lungs and out again.

We need large volumes of air to carry oxygen to our blood cells, which circulate through our bodies. These mobile messengers deliver oxygen and nutrients to every cell, organ, tissue, and muscle in our bodies. On the return trip, our blood cells carry carbon dioxide (a waste byproduct of our bodies) to the lungs, which, in turn, expel it in our exhalation. Breathing helps to regulate our heart rate and keep a constant supply of fuel going to our organs.

Too little oxygen causes drowsiness, fatigue, muscle aches, and stiffness. In a dominolike effect, long periods of sitting without occasional deep breathing cause poor circulation, and poor circulation and poor oxygen exchange, in turn, cause poor performance and inattention—all this because of improper and inadequate intake of air.

Poor sitting or sleeping positions inhibit good breathing. So, in order to insure an adequate supply of air to our bodies, we need to practice good posture (good balance) and deep breathing exercises, and do rigorous activity on a regular basis. By adding these elements to our routines, we allow our lungs to fully expand and contract with each and every breath, and thereby foster healthy respiratory and circulatory systems.

FLOW AND FLUIDS IN TRUCKS AND HUMANS

Numerous fluids are required for a truck's optimum operation. There is antifreeze, brake fluid, fuel, grease, oil, power-steering fluid, transmission fluid, windshield-washer fluid, and water. Regardless of which it is, if it runs out, that system will be compromised. Without water, an engine would quickly overheat and break down. Without brake fluids, you risk a disaster. Without oil, the engine would sieze up and grind to a dismal halt. Good vehicle care requires that all fluids be kept clean and full.

Of all the fluids on the planet, water is the most important one for us humans. There is more to water weight than that occasional bloating you might feel after a night eating buttered popcorn and salted peanuts. *Most* of your body is water. Plain and simple: 90 percent of your blood, 75 percent of your muscles, and 60 percent of your body overall is water.

Even without working up a sweat, just living your daily life causes your body to perspire. In other words, even when you aren't visibly sweating, you are sweating because, for example, the air around you pulls water from your body's largest organ, your skin, and your clothes absorb water from your body. If you are breathing, you are perspiring.

You might say, "I drink when I'm thirsty." But, when you are thirsty, it's too late, you are already dehydrated. Unlike a truck, you can keep moving around while you are dehydrated, but your body has to make up the water somewhere. So it drains water from your blood, muscles, and tissues, and when this happens, your heart has to work harder because thick blood is more difficult to pump. Dehydration can, again in a dominolike effect (like so many of our poor health habits), cause heart disease, high cholesterol, and hypertension.

Besides making up the vast majority of your body's weight, water has very important functions. It is the primary component in keeping other fluids and systems in your body, like the synovial and lymphatic fluids, functioning properly. The synovial fluid is the liquid that floats around most of the joints in your body, allowing them free movement. The lymphatic system provides your body with its best defense against bacterial and viral infections. Lymphatic fluid is found between your tissues and red blood cells and aids in ridding your body of toxins. When your body is dehydrated, these systems do not work very well and you can become bloated, stiff, or sore.

Water is also essential for waste management. It helps the colon, kidney, liver, stomach, and so on, to function, and it is what carries your body's waste to its final destination. Without water, this process of elimination is just that much harder, and, in fact, lack of water causes toxins and other waste products to build up in the body and significantly diminish health and well-being over time.

A good rule of thumb for water consumption is one-half ounce of water for every pound of body weight. If you weigh 180 pounds you should consume approximately 90 ounces of water every day, especially if you must physically exert yourself. Drinking that much water (eleven full water glasses, fewer if you weigh less) may seem impossible, but try working yourself into the routine and you could be pleasantly surprised at how natural it becomes. If you have questions about your water intake, be sure to contact your healthcare professional.

Let's figure that on an average day you drink two cups of coffee, one carbonated beverage, a glass of water, two iced teas, and maybe a couple of cocktails. Since that all adds up to approximately 88 ounces, you can see how it is possible to consume that much fluid without bursting or spending your life on the toilet. However, out of all of those beverages, the only one that is essential for keeping fit and healthy is water. Alcohol and caffeine have the reverse effect of water; they actually dehydrate your body. And carbonated beverages are prepared by injecting carbon dioxide into a drink. Carbon dioxide is a waste product of breathing and, as such, the body is happy to get rid of it by expelling it from the lungs when we exhale. Think about that for a few minutes the next time you pop a can of soda.

FLOW AND EXHAUST IN TRUCKS AND HUMANS

Engines burn fuel and a fully functioning exhaust system blows the waste out the tail pipe or vertical stack. In a truck, the waste consists of gases, fluids, and solids. The gases are carbon dioxide and carbon monoxide, poison to you and me. There is usually also water vapor that must be expelled from the combustion chamber, as well as ash, soot, and sulfur.

Plugged or obstructed exhaust systems can cause waste products to back up into the engine, thus making it work harder, and wasting fuel in the process. A harder working engine ages quicker, making a twofold economic impact: decreased fuel economy and decreased vehicle longevity. Conversely, a clean, efficient exhaust system promotes cost savings and extends life.

Like a truck with its gas, fluid, and solid waste, elimination of the body's byproducts is essential to health and physical efficiency. We've discussed the lungs and their role in eliminating carbon dioxide from the body. That is one phase of metabolism. Another phase is the digestive tract, which not only carries nutrients to various parts of the body through absorption, but also includes the body's main exhaust system for fluid and solid waste.

Similar to a truck, if the body's exhaust system is partially or completely clogged, the waste backs up with no place to go. When this happens, your body has to absorb the waste and store it in your tissues, organs, and muscles. As a result, your body becomes toxic, causing illness, fatigue, strain, lowered performance, and premature aging. More energy is required to complete tasks, with fewer reserves to accomplish them. Experts vary in their opinions about the frequency of bowel elimination, but the average is considered to be one to three times per day, ideally of well-formed stools.

A healthy digestive tract is essential for proper absorption of the nutrients needed to build a robust immune system and an energy-filled lifestyle. Eating healthy food, drinking sufficient fresh, pure water, applying effective stress-management techniques, and doing regular exercise goes a long way toward keeping your digestive tract healthy.

FLOW AND LUBRICATION IN TRUCKS AND HUMANS

Axles, drive shaft, gears, pistons, and wheels—the list is lengthy when it comes to truck parts. When the engine is running and the vehicle is moving, these parts churn, turn, and roll, time after time. Oil and other lubricants are distributed through the lubrication system to keep these machine parts from rubbing directly together, allowing them to turn or glide on a thin film of lubricant, and thereby reducing the amount of friction that builds up between the working parts. Reduced friction extends the life of the parts and increases the truck's efficiency. If the lubricants are allowed to run out, there will soon be excessive abrasion, friction, heat, and grinding. Those conditions make engine parts work harder to move, requiring more energy (fuel) to move them, with the end result being that the vehicle wears out faster.

Oil also cleans the engine. Oil streams through the running engine and picks up debris, such as dust, dirt, carbon, and flakes of worn metal. The smallest particles are caught in the oil filter, while the larger ones settle at the bottom of the oil pan. Frequent oil changes and filter replacement are essential to good engine maintenance because, once the oil is dirty, it fails to clean the engine. It begins, instead, to leave more residue behind in the engine with each pass through it, eventually causing damage to its moving parts.

When an engine is running, a thin layer of oil between the pistons and the cylinder walls prevents a loss of pressure. The power of combustion delivers a forceful push against the piston, which then sends maximum power to the drive shaft and wheels. If the layer of oil is absent, much of the power is lost, and the engine must work harder to move the vehicle. This reduces the life of the engine and other parts of the vehicle.

Another important function of oil is to protect the engines from corrosion, erosion, and rust. It also acts as a shock absorber between parts as they transfer the power of the engine. Regular oil changes and lubrication are essential to prolonging the life and maximizing the power of a truck.

Skeletal parts, such as bones, discs, and joints, can be directly related to the mechanical metal parts of a truck as they too require lubrication to work well and feel good, as do eyes and ligaments.

Bone rubbing against bone increases abrasion, friction, grinding, and heat, causing stiffness, swelling, and severe pain in the joint. Unlike trucks, we cannot go to a Lube & Tube and have our synovial fluid (joint oil) replenished; we must maintain it ourselves. Inactivity and dehydration decrease the amount of lubrication in our bodies, and also decrease the viscosity, or thickness, of the synovial fluid. Here's an easy solution: move those joints regularly through their total range of motion, eat a healthy diet, and drink plenty of water. Movement and stretching make the ligaments, muscles, and tendons more elastic. Flexible joints make it easier to breathe properly, maintain proper postures, and just plain move, plus they decrease your chances of injury.

FLOW AND WELL-BEING

Air and fluids are continuously moving in, around, and through the body, even when it is stationary. The flow of air and fluids is essential for optimum physical health and structural longevity. All body movements, postures, and activities, or lack of activity, directly affect flow, and thus impact various aspects of short- and long-term physical health and well-being, including, of course, aging.

BREATHE IN

The flow of air is first taken in through the nostrils and mouth and is transported into and out of the lungs. The structural home of the lungs is the rib cage, and its position in relation to the rest of the body has a great deal of influence over the rate and ease of airflow.

Slump forward in your chair and hold your head down. Breathe in, and let it out. Now assume a correct posture. Put the curve in your lower back forward, rock your rib cage so your shoulders are over your hips, and hold your head in a good posture. Take another breath in and let it out. In this proper posture, you will notice that it is easier to breathe in and out and notice also that you are able to increase the volume of air you breathe in and out.

Your body is designed to take in as much oxygen as necessary to carry on the functions that are required of it. Your job as the owner of that body is to maintain it in a position that allows for good airflow. When the upper part of the rib cage is slumped forward, the dynamics of air intake are altered and oxygen intake is diminished. Breathing air in and out of the body also influences your heart rate and the level of blood circulation throughout your body.

Posture affects airflow during all sitting, standing, and sleeping activities. If you sleep curled up in a ball, chances are your body will go through periods of shallow breathing. You should instead be in a good posture that encourages the intake of refreshing oxygen and the exhalation of carbon dioxide and other waste products that are byproducts of body metabolism.

THE FLOW OF FLUIDS

Fluids flow throughout your body, nourishing and bathing virtually every cell in it, at the same time they are removing waste products from it. Any disruption in the flow of any fluids, like blood, inhibits the intake of nutrients by the cells and the washing away of cellular waste products, such as lactic acid and protein debris.

In addition to the circulatory system, there is the lymphatic fluid system. Lymphatic fluid is found between the cells and tissues of the body where it helps clean and drain away cellular waste products. Along with the circulatory system, the lymphatic system provides a way for white blood cells and other immune system cells to defend the body against viral and bacterial invasion. When you are active, you stimulate the lymphatic fluid flow.

There is also synovial fluid, which flows around most of the joints of the body and acts as a lubricant to improve the efficient movement of your bones and reduce friction. To remain nourished and get replenished, this fluid depends on the movement of the two bones that make up a joint. When there is decreased movement between the bones that meet to form a joint, this synovial fluid can change its character and become less lubricating, actually increasing the friction between the bones. If that happens, the joint will become progressively stiffer and more difficult to move. Much like blinking your eyes keeps the eyeballs moist and lubricated, the movement of your body is its own automatic lubricating system for joints. Strengthening activities and full range of movement help keep your joints moving efficiently, and also promote elasticity in muscles and ligaments.

The stiffening of a joint can be a gradual process and can ultimately contribute to stiffness of movement and varying degrees of attachment between the bones. If you wrap your shoulder in a sling to immobilize it for twenty-four hours, it is very stiff and sore when you start to move it again. This stiffness is, in part, caused by a decrease in both blood and synovial fluid flow in the joint, ligaments, and muscles of the shoulder.

In addition, if the lubricant between the bones restricts the movement of the bones, the muscles have to work harder to move and this consumes more energy. The best way to promote an optimum flow of fluid around the joints is to do regular exercise and stretching, which will help maintain the joints in good positions and will allow them to move easily through their total range of motion.

YOUR SPINE AND DISCS

The discs, or cushions between the vertebrae of the spine, are more than 80 percent water, which is part of the reason why they are such good shock absorbers. When the spine is optimally aligned in its s-shaped configuration, the pressure on the discs is at a normal level. However, if the lower back loses its curve by becoming flattened, pressures on the discs automatically increase about 50 percent.

As with other joints, in order to remain healthy, nourished, and fully functional, each disc must have fluids flowing in and out of it on a regular basis. And each disc depends on movement to push these fluids out and pull them back in.

If, however, you assume postures and perform activities that reshape your back away from its natural, s-shaped position, there will be increased pressure on the discs to move fluid out. Sitting in a poorly fitted chair every day is a common example of this. If there is inadequate movement of the vertebrae, and your body's posture does not allow an equal amount of fluid to move back in, there will be a gradual migration of fluid out of the disc, which will cause the disc to become thin and age prematurely.

The weight-bearing and shock-absorbing aspects of the discs between the vertebrae are part of the body's original design and can withstand a great deal of pressure. But when the discs are compressed due to poor long-term posture and poor repetitive movements, they are more likely to develop problems and age prematurely. Take, for example, the long-distance truck driver whose back becomes a human shock absorber, mile after mile, bouncing around in the cab of the truck. If this long-haul driver has optimum posture, he or she can actually avoid absorbing the road and engine shock, and can end the trip quite comfortably, with far less wear and tear on the discs.

LET THE GOOD TIMES FLOW

Good body positioning and movements assist flow. For example, the tensing and relaxing actions of muscles squeeze blood through them and encourage its general circulation. This tensing/relaxing movement also stimulates the lymphatic flow.

In addition to air and fluid movement, flow can also be considered in body movement. Have you ever watched someone who has mastered a sport or a special skill use the flow of movement to accomplish such activities as a perfect dance performance, playing a game of golf with precision and skill, or navigating a racing car deftly through the pack? Those performing these feats so skillfully seem to work with minimum effort and thought, whereas beginners in the same activities will have jerky, awkward movements and, often, poor postures. Masters at a given task have a physical flow, or pattern of movement, that is more energy efficient and less harmful to the body. Like them, you can learn to master good posture and improve your body's flow. All it takes is practice.

Appropriate movements can stimulate air and fluid flow in the body. In addition, by stimulating airflow through deep breathing, especially in good postural positions, you stimulate fluid flow and the proper movement of the rib cage and upper body.

Closed or tight angles in the body and joints decrease flow. If, for example, you pull your knees up toward your chest, you decrease flow through the knees and hips and force the lower-back curve to reverse. While this position does provide some stretching and variety, if done excessively and repetitiously, it will eventually inhibit flow. The same is true for tight or closed fist, wrist, elbow, or shoulder positions, such as sleeping curled up in a ball, keyboarding with wrists tilted to the side of the little finger, or typing from too high a position.

The flow of fluids, including blood and synovial fluids, and fluids in and out of the discs, encourages nourishment and the continued ability to physically perform body movements. Ligaments and tendons, which work in coordination with the muscles, offer support and encourage safe movement, but to do the job well, they require good fluid and body-movement flow to remain strong, elastic, and healthy.

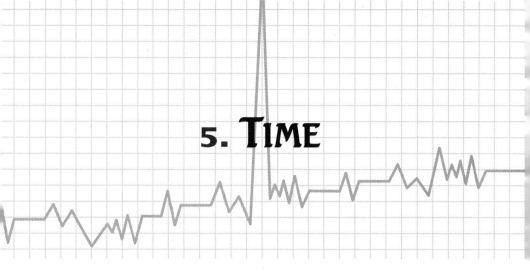

5. TIME

Time is technically defined as a nonspacial continuum in which events occur in apparently irreversible succession from the past through the present to the future.

Although time is certainly one of the most discussed phenomena in contemporary life, and seems to be blamed for a great deal of the stress in our lives, it is actually neutral and neither a friend nor an enemy. Rather it's what we do and don't do with our time that makes for its beneficial or detrimental effects on our bodies.

Time itself does not judge, but we can use time to evaluate our current condition and how we got there. Time is similar to an anchor in that it drives your predominant postures, movements, activities, and habits into your form. Time is also like a magnifying glass in which the negative abuses and deficiencies, as well as the positive actions and habits, become more and more pronounced.

Time can be used to better manage body habits, and to change your current balance, form, and flow into a more desirable state of health and well-being. You spin this day into the next, and the next, and, as you tunnel through your life, your habits are often the central factors in determining your physical health or lack of it.

You can pull yourself out of a downward spiral at any given time. Examine your habits, your surroundings, and the degree to which you physically interact with your surroundings, to gain insights into the path you are traveling and into what your ultimate physical destiny is likely to be. As you travel through time in your life, this introspection can provide you with the best opportunity for making any changes necessary to create a much more desirable destiny.

THE FIRST STEP

Momentum is already propelling your collective habits through time to a relatively predictable outcome.

To start taking control of your time, first determine the path you are now on and become aware of your own physical condition. Think about why you do the things you do. In cognitive learning, you begin by bringing information into your awareness, and you study it as it practically applies to yourself, and then it becomes much easier to make substantial and lasting changes in your life. For example, many times our habits are formed from learned behavior, social pressure, media conditioning, fear of change, and inertia. You can change these habits by first determining what you want your destiny to be, and then deciding what changes must be made. In reality, you do not need to adopt perfect posture all day and night every day. Keep your out-of-balance or slumped postures in perspective with your positive postures. Take the appropriate time to counteract the negative influences with stretching and breathing.

AGELESS/TIMELESS

It is difficult to talk about time without also discussing age, as age does represent the amount of time we have spent thus far in our lives. There are two aspects of age. The first, of course, is chronological age—how old you are in number of years. The second in physiological age—how old your body is in a biomedical sense. The two are not necessarily the same. Someone could, on one hand, be fifty-six-years-old chronologically, but have the body of a forty-five-year-old. A hard-living twenty-eight-year-old could, on the other hand, have the physiological body of fifty-year-old. You just have to attend your high school class reunions to see the phenomenon of this variant in action.

In my active practice, it is common to see people who are physiologically beyond their chronological age. Yet there are also many times that I see people who seem to be physiologically much younger. The components of youthful physiological age include:

➤ Good muscle tone;

➤ A desire to obtain and maintain appropriate postures in a more relaxed and less rigid manner;

➤ Good flexibility both in forward, backward, side-to-side, and rotation movements throughout the joints of the body;

➤ Enough stamina and physical conditioning to sustain the activities of daily living;

➤ A positive attitude and outlook on life; and

➤ Habits that encourage optimum balance, form, and flow.

The components of a body that has physiologically aged beyond its chronological time include:

➤ Chronically tight, tense, imbalanced muscles;

➤ An inability to hold and maintain optimum positions and postures;

➤ Shallow breathing;

➤ Restricted body movements, such as slumping postures arising from poor self-esteem, or depression, or from being forced to sit in a chair that doesn't fit properly;

➤ A pessimistic attitude; and

➤ Poor family or social support systems, and an inability to integrate and maintain positive habits.

6. REPETITION, FORCE, AND FLEXIBILITY

Repetition is the act, process, or instance of doing, experiencing, or producing something again and again.

Repetition is crucial to any activity you want to get better at, whether it is ice skating or ice sculpting. Repetition is what allows the hammer to drive a large nail through hardwood, or allows a small ax to cut through a huge tree. Repetition reinforces habits, both physically and through the brain and nervous system, that consciously or subconsciously direct your movements. Repetition is what trains your habits to either change or perpetuate their form.

Repetition makes habits and movements become second nature and get programmed into your brain and nervous system. Repetition of habits then carries on without your awareness so you can concentrate elsewhere. Repetition is like practicing the piano, the more you practice, the better you get. By the same token, the more you slump over your desk, the more you *will* slump over your desk.

The more frequently you repeat an activity, the more deeply embedded the neurological pathways that govern the actions from your brain through your nervous system become, pathways that tell the different muscle groups and other structures of your body what to do. In time, repetition magnifies the effect of your habits on your body.

With each repetition of an activity (a golf swing, a ballet position, a scale on the trumpet), you are programming your nervous system to respond in a specific way with less and less conscious awareness. The way to break established poor habits and adopt better ones is to first become aware of the habits. Decide what to change, and why, then use repetition and time to reprogram your actions into habits.

DRIP, DRIP, DRIP

Repetition is also what allows water to erode rock. You can use this powerful phenomenon to your advantage, but it can also work against you. Because repetition of activities becomes second nature so quickly, in order for you to change it, is essential that you become aware of what your body is repetitively doing that is harmful to it.

Repetition can work with time to create vibrant health or declining health. There is also an impact on the system depending on whether the repetition is forced or relaxed. Forced, or tense, repetition of a negative habit, for example, adversely affects the body at a greater rate than a relaxed repetition of that same negative habit. Repetition of movement and habits can include large movements, such as getting in and out of a car, or small movements, such as keyboarding on a computer. It can include high-force activities, such as digging dirt in your garden or lifting heavy objects, or low-force activity, such as bending your head forward to read a book.

As with time, you can use repetition to your advantage once you have identified what repetition of the negative habits is doing to your body and your health. By modifying those harmful habits and the number of times they are repeated, they will start to work as they were meant to, more in line with the design of your body.

FORCE

Force is the capacity to do work or cause physical change.

Force is used in many ways, and can either be an ally or an adversary depending on how you use it. Force can be harnessed to create intentional resistance so you can increase your physical condition and endurance, as in proper weightlifting workouts to increase your strength; running on an inclined treadmill to improve your cardiovascular condition; or properly performing manual labor to improve your capacity for work. In addition, properly using force in exercises stretches bones and muscles. Conversely, if you don't use proper force in your daily activities, exercise included, then your muscles and bones can atrophy. In these cases, the proper use of force against resistance is beneficial to you.

Misusing force can be very harmful, as for example, lifting a heavy box incorrectly, shoveling snow with a poor technique, or sitting slumped over the kitchen table reading the newspaper for a hour. In these examples, force causes your body to resist in a way that has harmful consequences. The force itself is neither positive nor negative, but how it is applied to your body determines what type of impact it has. You can make that choice. Take the example of a motor vehicle driver who experiences the repetitive force of vibration. If that person is sitting in an optimum state of balance, with the normal spinal curves intact, then the spine acts as a shock absorber and no undue pressure builds up in the body. Conversely, if you slump while driving or riding in a vehicle, pressure quickly builds in your back because you are reducing your body's shock-absorbing ability. When encountering stress, if the force is met with too much resistance and given too much importance (or weight), then there is a negative, tensing effect that accumulates over time. Recognize force as a phenomenon that needs to be respected, but one you can learn to apply to your advantage.

FLEXIBILITY

Flexibility is the quality of being adaptable and responsive to change, or of being pliable and able to be bent or flexed.

Flexibility is another fundamental that has a double meaning. Healthy and happy people of all ages exhibit flexibility in body movements, but, as we get older, maintaining this becomes increasingly important. The yogis have a saying that you are as young as your spine is flexible.

Dr. Grant Donovan of Australia studied people in their eighties and nineties with no histories of chronic illness and he made several interesting observations. First, he indicated that, although these people were not necessarily formally well-educated, they loved to learn. Also, when they woke up in the morning, they looked forward to what they would be doing that day, and generally had positive expectations. In addition, he noted they had very good joint mobility. Which came first? Did the good joint mobility cause the healthy longevity and positive attitude, or was it the other way around? I suspect these people worked on the flexibility of their bodies and minds by virtue of the habits they acquired. Again and again, we see people who suffer serious injury to their backs. They lose flexibility, experience pain, and cannot do the activities they feel compelled to do or want to do; what invariably follows is stress, anxiety, and depression. This is why attention to flexibility of both body and mind are essential during periods of stress, recovery from injury, and throughout daily life.

7. ANATOMY FOR A LIFETIME

Remember this concept and you will save yourself much misery and regret: Whenever imbalance disturbs flow through repetition and over time, your form will be changed in a negative manner; whenever you change balance positively and flow is restored, then time and repetition will likewise make a positive change in your form.

The basic fundamentals of balance, form, flow, time, and repetition can now be applied to virtually every activity or condition in life. You can use these basic fundamentals as the lens through which you view the most advantageous way of pursuing an activity aimed at enhancing your short-term and long-term health and well-being.

When considering balance, visualize your physical body in its space, with its many levers, fulcrums, and pulleys, so you can select the balanced positions and movements that are most appropriate and comfortable for you and your activities.

Always consider that balance and counterbalance create a situation in which less exertion is needed, and in which the action performed is the one most suited to the activity. Think about action and counteraction, pushing and pulling, lifting and bending—allowing many things in your environment to work with you to create actions and counteractions for a more artful performance of your actions.

We suggest you look at the figures in this book again and again to enhance your understanding of new ways to do everyday things. This process of self-discovery can be enlightening and exhilarating. Once you have started to make the changes, the momentum will increase and will help you continue to make further and even more helpful improvements.

When considering form, always keep in mind your unique physical shape and contour. Do not judge your present form, even if you wish it were a little smaller here or a little longer there. Consider what your current form actually is when taking steps to make your surroundings, such as your living areas, your workplace, or your vehicle, fit you better.

In addition to your unique contour, size, and shape, you should also keep your current physical condition in mind. Are you recovering from an injury or strain of some type? Are you receiving treatment for a certain condition? If so, then keep this in mind as you are making changes. If you have any questions about changes you could make regarding your health, always consult your healthcare providers for assistance.

For example, you might have scoliosis, a sideways curve to the spine. If you have this curvature of the spine, you need to create a unique fit between your own body and your environment, and it may be different from the fit for someone who doesn't have scoliosis, but you can, nevertheless, still make things fit more exactly for you.

When considering the best fit between you and your environment, your mission is twofold: to fit in your present form and, if necessary, to change the fit through time and repetition to one that is more desirable. Whatever you've been doing up to now has contributed to who and what you presently are. Make an accurate assessment of where you are, and use the examples in this book to actually reverse the aging effects that have started.

Consider any conditions that may make one side of your body fit differently into your surroundings than the other side. Some things in life just aren't in balance. You may have acquired imbalances from one-sided physical activities like tennis and golf or, in pre-backpack days, from carrying schoolbooks on one hip. Acquired imbalances can also be a product of habits and activities related to work, home, or leisure. Your approach to these activities can be modified to become more balanced by adding counter stretches and activities to neutralize the imbalanced actions.

Most of us have been unknowingly training our bodies to be in various states of imbalance. You can stop those actions from having detrimental effects on you. You can take charge and make changes that work for you. You can either change your mind to change your actions, movements, and habits, or change some habits to see if it is worthwhile to change your mind and make more changes.

The physics of nature indicate that balance is a desirable state for longevity. The degree to which you can better achieve balance in certain areas of your physical surroundings, your movements, and your habit patterns is the degree to which you conserve energy, reduce strain, and promote longevity.

After you've viewed an activity through the lens of balance and form, look at the different systems of flow we've discussed so far.

➤ Flow of oxygen: in with the good and out with the bad;

➤ Flow of blood: red cells—the nutrients and cleansers; white cells—the immune defenses;

➤ Hormones: the system regulators;

➤ Lymphatic fluids: transporters between tissues and blood;

➤ Movement: flow of physical activity;

➤ Spinal discs: essential in and out flow, balance, shock absorption; and

➤ Synovial fluids: joint lubricators.

Time and repetition drive balance and flow into your form. In order to change your form, balance, postures, and activities, and to stimulate flow, use time and repetition to make your changes real.

In the process of change, time becomes your anchor. Time will set balance, form, and flow into one of two paths: a movement toward declining health, or a process of continually renewing to revitalize your health and well-being for the long-term.

Repetition trains your body for balance, form, and flow. If your repetitions are beneficial to your physical system, you can train your body to your advantage. However, repetitions that take away from your proper balance, form, and flow cause you to drift away from optimum states that are within your reach.

THE PSYCHOLOGY OF SLUMPING

We slump for a number of psychological and physical reasons. Knowing why we slump is the first step toward changing our posture. Here are some of the reasons:

➤ **Poor self-esteem.** If you don't feel good about yourself, chances are you will not carry yourself proudly and erect.

➤ **Depression or anxiety.** These states of mind and body come with a number of outward symptoms. Slumping is often one of them.

➤ **Hiding to camouflage physical development** (particularly in adolescence and into adulthood). Teenage boys, for example, who are going through rapid growth spurts, may be self-conscious about their increased height. Middle-aged people worry about spare tires, the old midriff bulge.

➤ **Showing off.** On the other hand, bodybuilders who are intent on showing off abdominal muscle definition (the "six-pack") will bend slightly forward as they flex their abdominal muscles. Such flexing alters their balance toward a slump. You can see examples of this on the covers of men and women's health magazines.

➤ **Peer group pressure.** It may seem cool to slump against the school lockers or hunch over the desks, but it doesn't have to turn into a habit.

➤ **Fatigue.** You're just plain tired from physical activity, lack of sleep, or other metabolic conditions.

➤ **Ill-fitting clothes.** Trying to maintain good posture in platform shoes is impossible. As is walking through an airport with a purse slung over one shoulder, a laptop in one hand, and the handle of a rolling suitcase in the other. Or trying to walk with a small child. There is no way you can hold the child's hand and stand up straight.

➤ **Stress and tension.** No explanation necessary.

➤ **Injuries to our bodies.** They may alter our ability to move in certain ways. And postoperatively, many cardiac patients, for example, resist standing up straight because they are afraid they will burst open their stitches.

➤ **Proper posture techniques.** You simply haven't learned them yet.

➤ **Family training.** We often mimic our parents' postures. This supposed unwritten, genetic code may actually be acquired, instead, by parroting our parents. If it is, once recognized, it can be changed.

➤ **Personal beliefs.** You know you slump, but you feel there's nothing you can do about it.

Yes, you *can* change. But these body postures will not change unless you pay attention to the key factors and make the adaptations work.

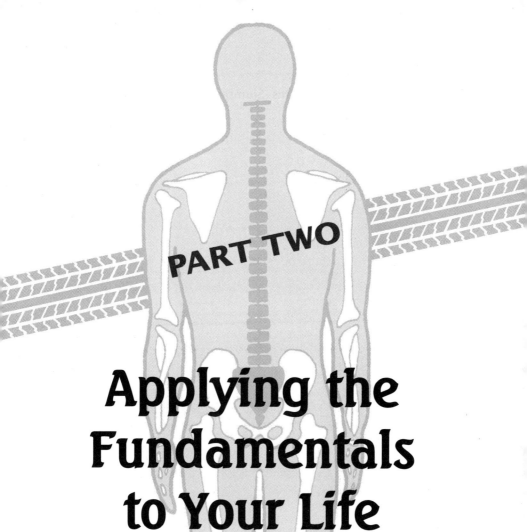

PART TWO

Applying the Fundamentals to Your Life

8. Seek Complete Recovery from Injury

When injury or strain occurs, causing tissue or cellular breakdown, there must be adequate circulation and airflow, plus an optimum amount of movement and flexibility in order to promote healing. If an activity causes strain and resulting tissue breakdown, then you must give your body a cycle of rest so it has time to repair itself and properly recondition the injured area to become strong, flexible, and healthy again.

Movement is an essential element of longevity because the body must be able to move through its designed ranges of motion regularly to maintain flexibility. If you lose your range of motion, you may experience increased friction in your joints, and, in a downward spiral, this can restrict your movement even further as time goes by.

The supportive tissues, such as ligaments and tendons, tend to conform to however the body is used. If the ligaments and tendons around a joint are not routinely stretched and put through range-of-motion movements, their full range of motion diminishes.

Do not let pain be your main indicator of recovery because it is often the first thing to get resolved in an injury. Returning to full balance, movement, strength, and comfort should be your goal.

DISCOVER RANGE OF MOTION

Let's check the range of motion in various parts of your body. Stand in front of a full-length mirror for this and, without pushing too hard, just check your ability to move comfortably through ranges of motion. Your goal is to see if you have symmetrical movement on each side of your body.

Check the figures in this chapter to determine if you are within normal

Lillian's Story

As Lillian stepped into a motorboat, it was suddenly shifted by waves and she was knocked over, injuring her back, which brought her to my office.

Lillian was an amazingly healthy eighty-six-year-old at the time and had lived a remarkably independent life. In terms of balance, form, and flow, her back was actually quite healthy and she therefore recovered quickly. I asked her why she thought her back had been so healthy. She told me that fifty-four years earlier, after she had given birth to her daughter, she'd had some back problems, and had begun doing several simple yet effective stretching exercises in the lower back and hip areas. The entire routine took just three to five minutes, she said, and she had done them twice a day ever since. Her rapid recovery from the boating injury proved their effectiveness and clearly demonstrated how the power of time and repetition was used to her advantage. Lillian also tells me she believes that people are as old as they talk themselves into being.

range. If one movement is much more restricted than the other, carefully review your work and home habits to determine whether or not frequent activities on one side only could be a source of your problem. If there is pain involved during any of the following movements of your neck, back, shoulders, arms, hands, legs, or feet, you should be professionally evaluated before getting involved in an exercise program.

Head Rotation: Rotate your head slowly to the right and take note where your head stops. Then turn your head to the left, noting where it stops (see Figure 8.1). Starting with your nose pointing straight forward, your head rotation is usually eighty degrees to the left and to the right.

Head Tilt: Tilt your head to the right, making sure you keep your nose straight ahead, then tilt it to the left (see Figure 8.2). Side tilting of the head is normally about forty-five degrees to the left and right.

Head/Neck Bending: Bend your head forward toward your chest (see Figure 8.3). Then slowly tilt your head backward (see Figure 8.4). Normally, a person can tilt his or her head far enough forward to touch the chin to the chest, and far enough backward to look at the ceiling directly above. If either of these movements makes you lightheaded or dizzy, seek professional assistance.

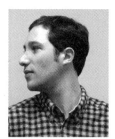 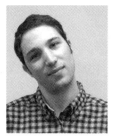 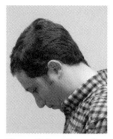 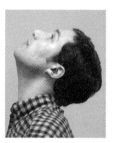

Figure 8.1. Normal head rotation.

Figure 8.2. Normal sideways tilting of the head and neck.

Figure 8.3. Neutral neck and head position; normal neck flexion.

Figure 8.4. Normal neck extension.

Back Bending: Bend forward at the waist. Without worrying about touching your toes, just bend as far as you can comfortably (see Figure 8.5). Now bend backward by tilting your head while bending your back slightly, being careful not to topple over (see Figure 8.6). If you bend forward about ninety degrees, and backward about thirty degrees, that's normal.

Side Bending: Bend at the waist, keeping your shoulders and hips straight forward. Bend to the right, then to the left (see Figure 8.7). Side bending is normally about thirty degrees in each direction.

Trunk Twisting: Keeping your hips facing forward, twist to the right, then to the left. Trunk rotation is normally about thirty degrees or more in each direction.

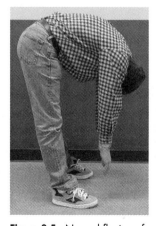 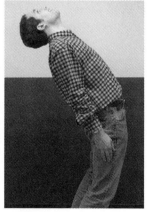 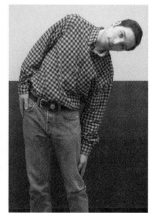

Figure 8.5. Normal flexion of the back.

Figure 8.6. Normal extension of the back.

Figure 8.7. Normal sideways tilting of the mid and lower back.

Other Body Parts: You should also rotate your shoulders, arms, wrists, fingers, legs, knees, ankles, and feet. The illustrations and guidelines for these are not included in this book, but check to see if you have unrestricted, painless, symmetrical motion in these joints.

My Story

One weekend, I took my son to Camp Kitaki. The kids were doing their camp activities and the parents, that sunny afternoon, found a big sandhill off to the side of the lake. We each attempted broad jumps off this hill, stretching like Olympic wanna-be's, and landing on the sand in a mock competition. Unfortunately, the previous several days of rain had compacted the sand underneath, so once the first few jumpers had landed in the dry top sand and kicked it away, the hard compacted sand underneath became the landing zone.

When it was my turn, I landed hard, unaware of the danger, and it felt as though a baseball bat had whacked me in the back. I lost all feeling from my mid-back down and couldn't move for a couple of minutes. I knew I was in trouble, but I slowly got up and stoically and carefully finished the afternoon's activities.

An x-ray the next day revealed a compression fracture at T11 in the thoracic part of the back, and I knew I was about to go through a recovery process that would shape the future of my back for the rest of my life. At forty-three, I wanted to heal completely so I could put this injury behind me and live another sixty healthy years with this back; this was the thought that drove my recovery process.

Pain became my coach and teacher. I listened to my body. When I wasn't comfortable, I could have taken a shortcut with medications, but I wanted to fully return the area to proper function. It would have been easy to succumb to the pain of a compression fracture, round my shoulders, slump and get on with life, but I was concerned about the long-term outcome.

In all my treatments, exercises, and activities, I always considered balance, form, and flow. Massage therapy helped ease my back pain, as did ultrasound therapy, and I kept moving safely about my daily activities. I was carefully monitored by my healthcare professionals who confirmed that I had sustained no nerve damage. I chose a careful yet aggressive treatment plan, and I was able to recover completely, with no slumping and no long-term degenerative effects so far.

—Dr. Scott W. Donkin

Any obvious restriction may mean that the joints have not been exercised for a long time, or it may be traced back to work or home habits, a previous injury, or surgery.

Movement enables flow. Every cell of your body depends upon proper nourishment and oxygen from breathing to remain healthy and vital for long periods of time. In fact, a French scientist conducted an experiment in which he isolated the heart tissue from a chicken embryo and immersed it in fluid that resembled normal blood for that tissue. He kept the heart tissue immersed in this fluid for twenty-eight years, changing the fluid daily, and for all that time, the tissue was alive and functioning well. When he stopped changing the fluid daily, the tissue cells died, leading him to theorize that the collection of waste products that are allowed to accumulate inside the cells contributed to the aging process and the demise of this tissue in his experiment.

We can learn from the example of the chicken heart. In the best of circumstances, our bodies have the potential for long and healthy life. All we have to do is provide those circumstances.

The flow of synovial fluid around and through the joints of the body is also diminished during periods of prolonged, repetitive, restricted movement. When the viscosity of the synovial fluid is diminished, the restriction that follows adversely affects the composition and function of the ligaments, muscles, and tendons that attach to the bones around the joints. On the other hand, regularly moving the joints through their full ranges of motion keeps them flexible.

When the spine is positioned differently from the way it was engineered, the pressures inside the discs increase, which then cause the fluid in the disc to flow outward, resulting in less movement of the vertebrae and less inflow of fluid into the disc. The disc then tends to dehydrate and thin, thus accelerating the degenerative changes that can occur later in life, and this is augmented by any previous injury and trauma to the discs and joints. That's why so many older people appear stooped or slumped. For them, time has taken its toll. This was not inevitable. Time and repetition have driven imbalance into their bodies.

LONG-TERM EFFECTS

The body attempts to heal or protect itself from damaging friction, inflammation, and irritation. In so doing, adhesions and scar tissue appear, the

David's Story

If you accept the notion that you can curtail certain movements, you're selling yourself short and will realize it later on. Too often, people will stop short in their recovery, especially from auto and work accidents, and will not heal properly. In any recovery, it's important to know your own highest capacity and strive for that in order to heal effectively.

David repaired boxcars at a railroad yard. One day, while fixing a car, a ram that was used to secure the car slipped and slammed a two by four into his head, crushing several of his facial bones, breaking his jaw, and giving him a whiplash injury in his neck.

Doctors had to reconfigure David's facial structure. His neck and back injuries were slow to heal and it took him a year to accommodate to changes in the seasons. Cold weather was particularly painful for him, but even when he felt the pain of the seasonal changes, David still went ahead and did the rehabilitative activities he was convinced were right for him. He had a goal. He wanted to return to his favorite pastime, car racing.

And now, three years later, he's enjoying it and his life in general. Doug taught me a lot about healing and recovery. For David, three years recovery was only a bump in the road of a long, healthy lifetime.

tissues thicken, and the result is a loss of function and movement. We have, in effect, adopted physical habits that contradict the body's natural course.

Suppose an injury occurs that strains or tears ligaments and muscles, or perhaps even breaks a bone. The body will take emergency action and begin the healing process immediately following the injury. Swelling occurs, as platelets, white blood cells, and other elements begin the healing by forming around the injured area. The injured tissues need to be challenged to heal safely yet early so they will resemble their former state and not develop scar tissue. That is why doctors who treat knee injuries start rehabilitation immediately and aggressively.

When healing from an injury, you should always keep balance, form, and flow in mind. Time and repetition of therapy and exercise will help determine the way the body recovers from the injury.

Is this less-than-optimum healing, or incomplete healing, a typical process of aging? It doesn't have to be. It is important for you to objectively review and understand what body balances you are doing every day:

➤ Do you sit all day?

➤ How often do you exercise?

➤ How do you feel at the end of the day?

Look at the following activities from the point of view of balance to understand, first of all, what needs to be changed:

➤ Do you reach with your right hand, or your left hand, all day at your job?

➤ Do you pick up your child with the same arm each time?

➤ Do you participate in a one-sided sport, such as golf or tennis?

Analyze the flow in each of your activities:

➤ Do any of your daily activities restrict your breathing?

➤ Can you move freely during the day, or are you required to sit in one spot?

Respect what your form is and decide how to fit it into your surroundings so that you can best achieve balance. Keep in mind that you can also improve your form by expanding your current abilities to achieve a better overall balance in your body.

➤ What can you modify at home or at work to achieve balance?

➤ What other daily activities restrict you, and what can you do about them?

Take a moment to reflect on what time and repetition have done in each of your activities and habits. Have your activities influenced the rest of your body? Will you be able to use time and repetition to effect changes in balance, form, and movement that make your activities work *for* you rather than contribute to, or magnify, current or future problems?

➤ Do you have chronic aches and pains?

➤ Are you tired by the end of the day?

➤ What activities can you add to your day to balance your body and life?

9. STRESS
WE ALL LIVE WITH IT

STRESS IN TRUCKS AND HUMANS

Stress on trucks can show up in tire wear, broken bolts on rims, structural damage to the body, frame, engine body, and transmission, and it can also result from improper maintenance or a collision.

Engine stress caused by air and oil filters, clogged fuel lines, or low fluid levels takes its toll on the machine. Stress can be caused by improper loading, or using the truck to do tasks for which it was not designed. Eventually, unattended stress will cause enough extensive damage for the truck to break down. To extend the life of the truck, it is important to take care of it through regular maintenance and appropriate handling.

With humans, understanding stress signs are key to keeping your body fit. Stress shows up through numerous symptoms, including anger, anxiety, attitude, digestive problems, fatigue, headache, high blood pressure, muscle tension, pain, strain, and worry. Unattended stress in your body and mind can cause enough compromising damage that your system will eventually break down, but, like trucks, regular, appropriate, preventive care of your body can extend its life.

THE DEFINITION OF STRESS

The word "stress" is an indication of pressure or tension. Originally, it was a technical term used for large structures and was described as a physical constraint that a mechanical piece, like a cable or an arch for a bridge, can endure. Today, although that engineering application still exists, the term stress is used more to describe a facet of our contemporary lifestyle. There are two reasons for that:

1. **The complexity of our existence.** Our present lifestyle is more complex than in previous times. Today, we process more information (bank and other access codes, social security numbers, telephone and fax numbers, as well as Internet address numbers), and the environment itself is more complex. For instance, it is stressful and challenging to navigate through and around a big metropolitan city during rush hour, with all the cloverleaves, access ramps, indication panels in the vehicle itself, not to mention the intense traffic. It has been found that the less control you have over the environment, the more anxious and stressed you feel—until, that is, you realize you must work with your environment rather than control it.

2. **The frequent and rapid number of changes.** Our lives are marked with many frequent changes happening faster than ever—job changes, changes in technology, changes in residency, personnel changes, and changes in friends and family. And studies have shown that stress levels are directly related to the quantity and rapidity of all these changes affecting us.

Today, stress and adapting to our environment are linked, and adapting to changes is an integral part of our definition of stress.

STRESS IN OUR DAILY LIVES

Stress invades virtually every aspect of our lives. We all live with stress. In fact, our cave-dwelling ancestors couldn't have survived without it. The problem is, in this technological age, we have to figure out how to control daily stress and make it work for us—not against us.

Here's how the stress response works: You're stuck in traffic, on a day your boss demanded a report ahead of schedule, and your teenage daughter just got her driver's license. Your body responds to the stressors: Your heart rate increases, transferring the flow of blood away from your digestive system to your arms, legs, and brain. You begin to breathe faster and perspire. Your body is preparing, naturally, for "fight or flight." You are gearing up for physical activity.

But, no, you're stuck in traffic, sitting in a car. You can't get to your office where your unfinished report looms, and you're wondering where your daughter is. If the prepared-for "fight or flight" activity is not realized or physically vented, then your body will increase metabolism in the muscles to vent that physical expression. If your muscles don't move through their range of motions and accomplish movement, the muscles will hold their tense position. In a sense, you're all stressed up with nowhere to go.

THE PHYSIOLOGY OF STRESSING

During a period of stress, your tense muscles contract, or increase, their tension, and they pull on the bones they are anchored to—pulling them together. The same phenomenon happens during prolonged out-of-balance postures.

Try this right now: Hold this book out at arm's length. How long does it take until you feel discomfort? Feel tense? Imagine another awkward position for yourself, such as slumping, and think what it is doing to the muscles in your back. Imagine what other awkward positions, besides slumping, can do.

Over time, this tension can actually result in permanently affixing an undesirable, out-of-balance position into your form. This is how poor posture is created. And, of course, there is a corresponding decrease in the ability of your body to move freely, even into more advantageous positions of balance.

Stress consumes a lot of energy. Your body works hard for absolutely nothing. Even worse, it works against itself. When your body expels energy in stationary tension, an increase in respiration may not be sufficient to fill the requirements of your increased metabolism so you become tired. You know the feeling: You're tired from a long day at work, and you've done absolutely no exercise, but you have been tense all day. This tension has created your fatigue.

Another good example is driving or riding in a vehicle for a long period of time. You're tense. You haven't vented your energy and you've become tired as a result.

Even more damaging effects come about through mental stress and your inability to release it. Your muscles become tense from stress, your flow of blood is lowered, your muscle's metabolism increases, along with your muscles' requirements for more oxygen and food. Because there is less blood and lymphatic flow through this area, there is a buildup of waste products that acts as an irritant to the muscles and decreases their ability to keep functioning at optimum healthy states. If the muscle tension occurs in the upper and mid-back, and in the muscles between the ribs, restricted breathing can result, additionally reducing the intake of oxygen.

Even if life is rosy for you, you could still be suffering from stress. Poor sitting postures combined with inactive muscles cause decreased circulation and decreased exchange of oxygen and nutrients in those muscles, which can cause irreparable damage. You can prevent the damage. Again, the key to eliminating this type of stress is through movement and breathing. Through flow.

When people are under stress, they often develop shallow breathing. Developing good deep-breathing techniques increases the amount of fresh oxygen taken into your body, and eliminates more carbon dioxide during exhalation, which can help to reduce the negative effects of stress.

ACCUMULATING STRESS

Let's look at saving money. You save money by investing in an interest-bearing account. Through the magic of compounding interest, your money grows in value over time and can provide a solid foundation for you and your family. Just like money in the bank, smart health habits can also help you build a solid, lasting foundation in your body.

If, on the other hand, you don't save any money, you may fail financially. Debt builds up, compounds negatively, and you find yourself trapped and unable to change the course of your finances. Similarly, your body can accumulate a debt of ill health, with poor habits contributing to the failure of your body's "account."

We all experience periods of stress, but if we do not take the time to counter those effects, tension and strain will accumulate and alter posture and form. And the resulting decreased flow can eventually become ingrained into our systems, negatively affecting our health and well-being.

STRESS AND PERFORMANCE

In 1906, two American researchers, Yerkes and Dodson, first pointed out what is well-known today: the relationship between the degree of activation and the success in performing a task at hand (at that time, the word stress was not yet in usage). They demonstrated a Double Inverted Curve of Stress versus Performance.

As it is with a car, where you should avoid underruning or overruning the engine, the optimal performances for people lie in the middle range of stimulation. With motor vehicles, the middle performance zone is engineered into the vehicle, but the human body has more options. We are capable of increasing or decreasing the optimal zone of performance by either increasing our mental and physical capacity, or decreasing it by doing nothing. This concept becomes very important in deciding how we can consciously shape our own destiny.

STRESS, ANXIETY, AND DEPRESSION

Generally, there is confusion regarding stress, anxiety, and depression. Stress is not a sickness, whereas anxiety or depression can be.

Here is an easy way to look at the differences:

Stress occurs when the signs that are complained about appear only in the presence of stressors. If the work is stressing, people will feel better during weekends and holidays when they are distanced from the stressors.

Anxiety occurs when the symptoms persist even away from the stressors. If the work is stressing, but the person is still concerned with the job during weekends or vacations, that person has internalized the stress and can produce it at a distance from the stressor.

Sometimes, what a person calls stress is in fact depression. The person becomes incapable of taking any action; almost everything seems difficult and insurmountable; feelings of acute tension, frustration, sadness, or discouragement are present. Stressed or anxious people are still involved in action and are capable of making the effort to adapt, but the depressed person gives up all efforts to fight and considers any attempt to regain some control over the environment unnecessary or impossible to achieve.

Although not usually the case, it is possible that these three phases can each occur in the same person, escalating from stress to anxiety to depression if that person is repeatedly exposed to too many important stressors.

SELYE GENERAL SYNDROME OF ADAPTATION

This rule is as follows: After exposure to an acute stressor, the human organism first receives the blow, then mobilizes resources (alarm phase), then enters a phase of resistance where all the mobilized physiological reactions are turned against the aggression. Afterward, there is a power drain when all the energy reserves get exhausted. Then recovery.

ECONOMIC DISTRESS

A 1993 study under the auspices of the Bureau International of Travail (B.I.T.) in Geneva, Switzerland, found that stress was one of the most important problems facing today's society. Stress, the report stated, can endanger physical and mental health, and can, furthermore, cost both companies and national economies a great deal in lost time and income.

In the United States alone, the cost of stress to industry is estimated at more than $200 billion a year in absenteeism, loss of productivity, health insurance, and outright medical costs. In Great Britain, the tab for stress approaches 10 percent of the Gross National Product.

STRESS MANAGEMENT

Countering Stress in the Body

You've heard this before, but it is so important that it's worth repeating. The best way to counter the stress that shows up in our muscles is through stretching, deep breathing, relaxing, and good body movements and balances. Time and repetition spent in counteracting the negative effects of stress have a cumulative beneficial effect. Repetition can steel the body against the stress reaction, and repetition of counter activities can actually change the course of your health and well-being for the better.

It's your choice. You can allow stress to magnify poor postures, compress good postures, and accentuate the negative aspects of time, or with the appropriate countermeasures, you can magnify the effects of improved flow of air and fluids, and improve your form.

Don't underestimate the power of a smile in stressful situations. Physiologically, it reduces some of the negative aspects of stress and gives you the opportunity to actually choose to have a positive outlook.

Preparing to Manage Stress

We all do some kind of stress management without even realizing it. Walking a few minutes to relax after a day's work or sharing confidences with a friend are both good examples of this, but we need to consciously do more to help ourselves and others.

By being better prepared for what to expect, people can learn to improve how they cope with stress. Stress managers and consultants have developed many excellent programs; we will detail an important one here.

Reacting to stress is as essential for survival as breathing and eating are. But, overreacting to stress or experiencing excessive stress will trigger negative consequences so it is important to manage stress efficiently.

Focusing on Health

In managing stress, good nutrition is essential for optimum health because overeating and other improper eating habits can trigger health problems and shorten life expectancy. It is better to keep our reactions to stress, as well as our eating patterns, within healthy limits for our bodies.

Focusing on Efficiency

There is an optimal individual threshold for a person to remain motivated and capable of peak performance. And there are a wide variety of stress management programs that focus on sports or specific occupations. Here are a couple of ways that you can manage stress:

1. **You can focus your action on the stressor.** Find a way to either keep from being exposed to the stressor or at least reduce your exposure to it if you cannot altogether eliminate the cause of the stress.

2. **You can focus on your reaction to the stress.** With this strategy, you manage your stress by countering or neutralizing your own reaction to the stressor.

Perhaps you realize that the stressor is only adding to your already being tense because you're overloaded at work, or you have personal or family matters worrying you. If this state of affairs is not to your liking, it it can be ameliorated if you choose to get your act together, get organized, take a walk, play a sport, or get in better shape overall, always remembering to keep some time available for your family and friends.

Different Approaches to Managing Stress

In order to implement these different stress management strategies, you can use one or several approaches, individually or together. Specifically, you can try the various methods of relaxation; the behavioral approach where you perform the activity and draw conclusions from that; the cognitive approach, which is the opposite—you learn about something first and then apply what you learned to what you do; or you can use stress moderators.

A stress management program can be composed of different ingredients. There is no one perfect stress management program, there are many different ones that vary according to the person and the stress symptoms, just as a diet is always best when tailored to the individual. Whichever method is chosen, it must be reasonable to you and be a validated approach.

Relaxation Is the Opposite of Stress

Relaxation response can be described as the opposite of a stress reaction. People using the relaxation plan were tested, and it was found that their reactions were exactly opposite to those normally experienced during times of stress. These reactions include:

➤ Reduced cardiac and respiratory responses;

➤ Lowered muscular tension;

➤ Warmer extremities;

➤ Lower blood pressure;

➤ Lower circulating catecholamine (adrenaline) levels; and

➤ Reduced activity of the limbic system (the part of the brain involved in emotions and preservation of the body).

All the above phenomenon are also observed in sleep, but during relaxation the person stays awake and can voluntarily interrupt the process at any time.

The relaxation reaction differs from the stress reaction in two major ways: 1) Relaxation is voluntary and the person must decide to do it, as the reaction to stress is spontaneous and involuntary; and 2) Relaxation must be learned in order to override our reactions to stress, which are ingrained.

In stress management, relaxation appears to be the most direct path to controlling the stress reaction because it can counteract any adverse physiological reactions to excessive stress.

Progressive Relaxation Technique

One very effective method for countering stress is through the Progressive Relaxation Technique. Progressive relaxation consists of alternately tensing and relaxing different groups of muscles, thus forcing you to focus on how it feels to relax. Here are the simple steps:

1. Sit on a comfortable chair, or lie on the floor with your feet against the wall, and close your eyes.

2. Make a tight fist with your hand, hold it for about five seconds and experience the tension.

3. Unclench and let the tension flow out, noting how it feels different to relax.

4. Do the same with your left hand and the muscles in your upper arms and shoulders.

5. Tense your neck, hold and relax, noting the feel of the relaxed tension.

6. Frown as hard as you can, and relax.

7. Smile as hard as you can, and relax (remember how it feels and be sure to use these muscles more than your frowning muscles).

8. Raise your toes (or push against the wall), feeling the leg tension, and relax. Again notice how the tension drains away.

9. Take a deep breath, feeling the tension in your chest. Exhale and relax. Breathe in again and hold, then exhale and concentrate on how calm you are.

10. Daydream about a peaceful, pleasant setting and enjoy it for a while.

11. Now count slowly to four and open your eyes. You'll be fully alert and relaxed.

Practicing this relaxation technique daily may initially take about twenty minutes, but the time will shorten as you become accustomed to it. If you do this exercise on a daily basis, you will benefit, not only in your work, but also in your general health and well-being.

From an S to C in 24 Hours

Let's look at a scenario for a day of typical working and leisure habits. In so doing, notice that most of our surroundings are not engineered to support the contour of our legs, hips, back, shoulders, arms, and neck.

- You wake up from a poor night's sleep on a mattress that's too soft and a pillow that twists your neck.

- You grab a quick breakfast and eat on the run.

- You shoehorn yourself into the driver's seat of your car. You slump forward to get closer to the steering wheel. Your knees are straight and locked.

- At work, your computer screen is to the left of your desk. You reach for your telephone on the right side, tip your left ear to your left shoulder to hold the phone and scribble notes at the same time. You wonder why your neck aches at the end of the day.

- Lunch is at a restaurant. You sit in a very uncomfortable booth. Every minute or two you rearrange your legs, trying to find a comfortable position. You never succeed.

- Back to work where you reach right for the phone and look left at the computer monitor.

- Leave work, lug a heavy briefcase three blocks from the office to your car, and throw it into the trunk.

- Stop at the grocery store on the way home. Push a heavy cart around the aisles. Stand in line to check out. Lug heavy grocery sacks up the steps. Reach high and low to put groceries away.

- Cook dinner in a kitchen where the countertop is too low for you, and eat dinner sitting on a barstool at the counter, legs dangling and back slumped forward.

- After dinner, you plop down on your couch and sink into the fluffy pillows.

- After a couple hours sleep crumpled up on the couch, your neck tilted back, mouth open, snoring, you drag yourself into your not-so-comfortable bed for yet another night of restless sleep.

The rest of this book is devoted to showing you how to get through your day and night, how to adjust your environment to your body, instead of the reverse, how to keep the S-curve in your spine and maintain balance, form, and flow, with time and repetition in everyday activities, so you do not have to be the victim of the pain-inducing C-curve.

MIND STRESS AND BODY STRESS

Trying to define the relationship between the mind and the body is a little like trying to figure out which came first, the chicken or the egg. And the same goes for trying to figure out what causes stress in the first place. At least, with stress, we can start with where it first manifests itself, in the mind or in the body, and proceed from there with the knowledge that a mental stress can reduce physical performance just as a physical stress can lower mental energy.

Recognizing the fact that we owe it to those who give us our paychecks to come to work fit and ready for a good day's work, we have to consider how everything we do in our personal downtime, including eating, drinking, and sleeping, will affect our performance on the job. Reciprocally, the quality of our day at work will affect our ability to enjoy, relax, and rejuvenate before returning to work the next day, and the next, and the next.

Many factors have an effect on the brain: alcohol, drugs, hunger, lack of sleep, medication, poor diet, and thirst, to name some, and all relate to how well your body functions, as do stress, fatigue, and improper posture. These are signs and symptoms you should learn to recognize so you can help your mind and body.

When your mind and body are healthy and have been well nourished, any job you take on will be easier to complete successfully. How can you keep your mind and body healthy? Simply by eating right, getting plenty of sleep, exercising regularly, and trying to avoid stressful situations, or at least minimizing them through any of the methods we have discussed here.

As your mind learns how to recognize the language of your body and tend to its needs, you will find the course of your life and your health improving immensely. You can't avoid stress entirely, so it's important to find an appropriate avenue to relieve it.

10. SITTING

THE ANATOMY OF SITTING

Sitting is not just about where your body meets the seat. It also includes the positioning of the entire body, from head to toes. The position of your chair can be likened to a shoe on your foot that must exactly fit its unique contours, forms, and arches in order to provide balance, and allow you to be supported while performing your tasks without giving your foot a second thought.

Look at your sitting form because you may have developed poor habits gradually and what may feel right to you now could in reality be biomechanically awkward. Form may be hard to see for this reason, but you can understand what your form is like by looking in the mirror, or at pictures, or by asking others. Ask a family member or a coworker to look at the pictures in this book and then observe your positions. You can do this with each other and it will help both of you make changes that will work better for you.

I admit, it is difficult to look at others to exemplify good postures, movements, and work habits because most of us have developed the same poor habits, and since the majority of us are doing it wrong, wrong looks normal. Most people (about 80 percent) are going to develop a back problem, if they don't already have one, and it is largely due to poor habits. Changing over to good habits may feel awkward at first, but change always does. Carefully study the figures in this book and seek assistance if needed.

Always seek professional healthcare advice if you have questions, or have any discomfort in your bones, joints, muscles, and nerves. Review the illustrations of correct posture in this book frequently. The longer you have had the poor habits that have created your form, the more time it will take to make those changes.

It is very important to understand patterns of flow in the sitting position. Airflow patterns are commonly forgotten, especially when an individual is concentrating on another task: the rib cage gets rocked forward, the legs are still, and there is an almost universal tendency to become a shallow breather in prolonged seated postures. Shallow breathing is not a positive activity because it reduces the amount of oxygen intake and decreases the amount of carbon dioxide and other metabolic waste products that get exhaled. This, in turn, contributes to fatigue, and decreases your concentration and your enjoyment of tasks.

Awkward positions, or fewer movements of the overall body, restrict the flow of blood through the legs and arms, especially when you are sedentary and your breathing is shallow. Have you ever found yourself sitting for a long period of time? Your heart rate and the amount of blood being pumped to your heart can slow down, thereby resulting in reduced nourishment to all areas of the body. Notice how quickly your feet become swollen and your shoes get tight after sitting for a while.

The movements of your legs, arms, and the rest of your body, by alternately relaxing and contracting your muscles, acts to squeeze blood back to your heart and stimulate your circulation. Movement is essential to flow. More open angles at the ankles, knees, hips, and elbows encourage flow, and the circulation of blood flowing around these angles gets decreased when the angle is increased. In other words, you can increase flow in your legs if your knees are not folded under you.

Being in sedentary positions over the years has an increasingly damaging effect on the flow of fluids around the joints of the body. In time, the increased friction it causes will limit your ability to move overall. This increased friction, combined with poor forward body positions and repetition can create inflammatory conditions and repetitive strain, which result in cumulative trauma disorders, such as carpal or tarsal tunnel syndrome, bursitis, and tendonitis.

The increased pressure in the discs caused by a poor forward sitting position can lead to premature degenerative changes in your body—particularly your spine that you rely on for support. Gradually, your balance, form, and flow may degenerate and to a great degree determine the destiny of your physical health and well-being. Conversely, it can provide a platform for making some of the most profound changes for the better in your physical health.

SITTING ON THE JOB

Heavy lifters aren't the only ones who suffer from a day's hard work. Millions of office workers and professional drivers are also the victims of aches and pains caused by the stress of sitting down too long, too awkwardly. We will specifically address sitting for drivers and passengers in Chapter 12, but for now, we will concentrate on general sitting, which drivers can also benefit from.

Millions of people who sit while they earn their living endure needless, excessive pain, stress, and strain as they perform their daily tasks (see Figure 10.1). Although these complaints are common, they are not normal, and they are definitely not necessary evils in today's high-tech society.

The good news is that you don't have to suffer while you sit (see Figure 10.2). You can alleviate many of the aches and pains associated with sedentary working by making adjustments to your work setting and by taking stress-reducing exercise breaks. Subtle body-posture changes and a chair with a good fit will make a substantial difference in how you feel and will allow you to concentrate more fully on your work.

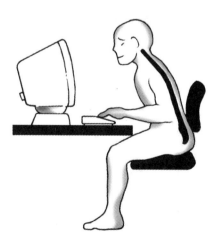 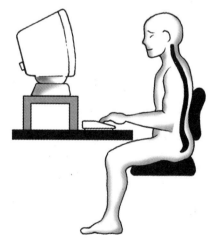

Figure 10.1. Poor seating adjustments and workstation arrangement often lead to increasingly poor posture, as well as pain, stiffness, and reduced performance.

Figure 10.2. Optimum seat adjustment and workstation arrangement encourage optimum postures.

COMMON PROBLEMS, SMART SOLUTIONS

Wrist

COMMON PROBLEM: Wrist pain, hand and finger pain, numbness, or tingling can result from improper positioning of your keyboard.

SMART SOLUTION: If you frequently use a keyboard, it is usually better to keep your elbows close to your body and your wrists parallel to the keyboard. By not bending forward, backward, inward, or outward, you reduce the strain on your wrists and forearm muscles, and ensure better positioning of your upper arms, shoulders, and neck. You can reduce wrist strain by avoiding the extension of your wrists and by preventing your wrists from pointing outward while keying.

Your keyboard and your mouse should be positioned so that you can hold your arms at a 90 to 100 degree angle, with your wrists in a neutral or "karate chop" position. Keyboards that are too high or too far away will alter your balance. If these can easily be moved closer, then your arms can be in a balanced position. If your arms have to extend out too far from your body to reach the keyboard, your posture suffers.

Eyestrain

COMMON PROBLEM: Eyestrain results from long hours at a computer or from visually intense work.

SMART SOLUTION: Reduce eyestrain by frequently changing your focus to an object far away, or by closing your eyes. Your eyes need frequent vision breaks to minimize strain.

Headaches

COMMON PROBLEM: Tension-type headaches can commonly be a result of tension, eyestrain, and poor posture.

SMART SOLUTION: Reduce your chances for headaches with proper posture and good lighting. Eliminate reflective glare on your computer monitor by rearranging work materials and equipment. Close the blinds or adjust the lighting.

Neck Pain

COMMON PROBLEM: Neck pain can result if you do repetitious movements, tilt your head forward for a long time, or perform one-sided head and neck turning (toward a computer monitor or colleague). Such tasks put extra pressure on the shock-absorbing discs between the vertebrae, which protect the nerves. This extra stress also affects the joints between the bones, and strains ligaments, muscles, and nerves. Over time, if this cause of neck pain is neglected, it can lead to a gradual, progressive erosion of the neck bones.

SMART SOLUTION: Reduce neck pain by adjusting your workstation to fit your body so your head is not unnecessarily tilted or rotated too far. Also, take periodic breaks and exercise your neck, shoulders, arms, and upper back to counteract the effects of head tilting. If you use the phone a lot, consider requesting a headset so you won't have to tilt your head while on the phone, especially if you need to use your hands to write or use the keyboard while you are on the phone.

Shoulders and Arms

COMMON PROBLEM: Shoulder and arm symptoms can result from arm positions and task postures that are unnatural to your body. Perhaps your files are just out of reach, and you have to strain to place files in your out basket. If your mouse is higher than your keyboard, then your arms must be in an extended position, and this can cause problems.

SMART SOLUTION: Align your body with your chair, your workstations, and your task to reduce the twisting and strain on your back, neck, and shoulders. Rearrange your office equipment to accommodate you, rather than your having to accommodate to your office.

If you cannot make a chair fit these parameters, then you can use cushions and wedges to retrofit your chair for your own body. Armrests, if you have them, should be high enough for you to rest your arm without altering your balance. If the armrest is too low, or too far away from you, you have to shift your body balance in order to reach it, and this is not beneficial to you. Keep in mind that the armrests should not interfere with your movements around your desk or keyboard if you use a computer.

Back Pain

COMMON PROBLEM: Back pain caused by unsupported sitting increases strain and fatigue.

SMART SOLUTION: Reduce back pain when sitting in your chair by placing your buttocks as close as possible to where the seat and backrest meet. Adjust the backrest and the height of the chair's seat pan so they fit the unique contours of your back and hips and allow you to sit comfortably erect. Use the backrest while working.

To derive the full benefits from the chair's backrest, you must place your hips so that your shoulders can move over your hips and allow your lower back to be curved forward. You may have to scoot your tailbone back into the corner of the chair where the backrest and seat pan meet.

The backrest of the chair should fit both the form and contour of your hips, your sides, your rib cage, and your back. Invariably we see, instead, that the backrest does not fit an individual's exact form, and is not positioned forward in the lower back, and the cushion does not fit the depth of curve of the lower back.

This support should be placed higher than most people have it in their workplace. Place the back of your hand and forearm across your lower back so you can feel its normal forming curve and then rock your rib cage into good position. If you visualize what this can be like in your own chair, you can do the same thing in your workplace.

Fatigue

COMMON PROBLEM: Fatigue is difficult to measure but is often described as feeling tired, lacking enthusiasm, or having no energy.

SMART SOLUTION: One answer to fatigue is exercise. Stretch and move during your scheduled breaks, and take several micro-breaks throughout the day.

Legs and Feet

COMMON PROBLEM: Leg and foot symptoms often result from poor blood flow through the legs because of lack of movement. If your chair's seat pan is raised too high, the resulting pressure on the backs of your thighs and bones of your pelvis can cut off the flow of blood.

SMART SOLUTION: Your chair height should allow you to plant your feet firmly on the floor or a footrest (even if your footrest is a thick phone book). It is essential to frequently flex and extend, and move your feet and legs in order to keep your blood flowing.

The form of your legs, from your feet to your knees, should determine the height of your chair's seat pan, just as the form and length of your thighs, from your knees to your hips, should determine the length of your seat pan. If the seat pan is too long, you won't be able to reach the back of your seat. If your seat pan is too short for your form, then you will feel uncomfortable in the chair and you will not be supported properly.

THE RIGHT SIT

As you position yourself for task-intensive work in your workplace, whether on the computer or with materials on your desk, keep in mind that your axis of vision should support good body position. The distance of the computer screen and other visual materials from your body is partly determined by your visual acuity and can have a substantial impact on your posture. Some people prefer the viewing screen away from their bodies, others like it closer. Only you can decide if you feel balanced in your workstation.

As you sit, your arms and legs, and your line of vision either act to pull the rest of your body out of balance or can help it achieve a balanced position. You can strive for appropriately balanced postures while performing these tasks:

1. Keyboarding and mousing;

2. Typing;

3. Writing and paper handling;

4. Talking and meeting; and

5. Driving.

Remember, however, it is not just the support from your external environment that is necessary. How you apply your body to complement the fit of your environment is also essential.

You can arrange items on your desk to fit your posture better. If you are in a conversation-oriented task that has you on the phone a lot or has you in discussions at meetings, you can lean back in your chair and allow the backrest of your chair to fit you better. The challenge of the chair's backrest, and this is true of any chair, is to actually fit into the contour and depth of the curve in your lower back. So moving your backrest into your body horizontally to support an upright vertical position requires an exact fit to your form and to the contour of your backrest.

Go ahead and arrange your workplace according to your posture as much as is practical and then begin working. If you find yourself always being pulled forward or out of balance, look at the way your workplace is configured. See if you can make any modifications. You may be extending your arm to use a mouse that is positioned too high. You might be looking at a document that is too low on your desk or trying to reposition around glare or reflections on your screen.

Next, look at your form. You may already be acclimated to old body postures and habits that have accumulated over time. Now may be an opportune time for you to make a transition and help your form change into a better-balanced position. If that's the case, then it is important for you to check particular areas that you find are being pulled out of balance. Check your flexibility in these areas and notice how your body stretches and moves through the normal ranges of movement.

TAKE A SIXTY-SECOND BREAK

Performing a physically and mentally demanding task requires intermittent rest breaks in order for the body to eliminate any accumulation of strain or irritation. I suggest you set up a cycle of resting and stretching to erase the effects of this strain. If there are areas in your workplace the you cannot fit into with your best position (for example, your workstation, the sales floor, the filing area), then pay particular attention to resting and counter-stretching. If some of your work tasks require you to turn your head more to the right, or bend your body more to the right during the day, make sure you incorporate stretches to the left to counteract that movement.

SIXTY-SECOND STAND-UP, PERK-UP BREAK

1. Stand up.

2. Kick off your shoes.

3. Rock back on your heels, then roll up on your toes.

4. Stand flat-footed.

5. Close your eyes, wiggle your hands and fingers.

6. Push your chest out and up like a soldier.

7. Breathe in deeply, slowly. Exhale. Do it again.

8. Smile.

9. Lift both shoulders toward your ears, and then push them backward. Try it one more time.

10. Relax your shoulders and arms.

11. Look toward the floor, then toward the ceiling.

12. Look straight ahead, then turn your head slowly to the right and to the left. Keep smiling!

13. Breathe in deeply, then exhale slowly.

14. As you sit down, aim your tailbone toward the place in the chair where the backrest and seat pan meet.

Here's what you just accomplished (all in just sixty seconds):

➤ You released the lock of your visually and mentally demanding tasks.

➤ You gave your buttocks, pelvis, and lower spine a break from bearing the entire weight of your upper body, and allowed your spine to assume its natural posture.

➤ You activated your lower leg muscles that stimulate the circulation of blood through your legs and back to your heart.

➤ You gave your eyes an essential vision break, allowing them to change focus.

➤ Deep breathing stretched and exercised your chest muscles and expanded your rib cage, which had become compressed as you slumped in your chair. At the same time, you refreshed your body with extra oxygen.

➤ You improved your posture by pushing your chest up and out.

➤ Smiling interrupted the stress cycle, allowing you to focus your attention on current tasks.

➤ Your neck and shoulder movements relieved the cumulative muscle tension and spinal restriction that occurs while performing prolonged sitting tasks.

➤ Sitting down properly allowed your body to achieve a more natural, healthier seated posture.

SITTING FOR COUCH POTATOES

The last thing people want to think about when finding a place to relax is how to best position their bodies. After all, relaxing is a time to do just that—nothing. Relaxing should give your body time to rejuvenate, so be careful not to let your S-curve become a pain-inducing C-curve.

Take a few minutes to set up your leisure environment so you can truly be comfortable and get proper support for your form. Start by taking a look at your current habits so you can make your leisure time work for you rather than against you.

Where do you go to relax?

LOUNGE LIZARDS BEWARE

If you have a recliner or lounge chair you like to lean back in, go ahead and lean back in it. Leaning back seems like a good way to take pressure off your body and allow it to rest and recuperate from the day. But the position of your body while you are in this restful pose is extremely important.

If your lounging posture is not balanced, but you are slumped forward instead, your body is conforming to an awkward configuration (see Figure 10.3). Like a left foot in a right shoe, this so-called restful position is actually working aggressively against your balance and form in the following ways:

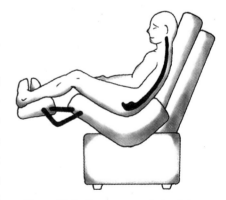

Figure 10.3. Poor support during leisure seating can add to the effects of poor postures in other areas of your life.

➤ Your lumbar spine causes your lower back to be flattened rather than curved forward;

➤ Your rib cage is rocked forward; and

➤ Your head is also tilted forward.

Reclining can take the pressure of gravity off your spine, but if you have to crank your head around to watch TV or to talk, then the position becomes counterproductive.

THE COUCH POTATO'S GUIDE TO CHOOSING A RECLINER

Being a full- or part-time couch potato isn't always easy. In fact, it can be downright hard on your lower back and neck. Improper couch potatoing will certainly cause long-range difficulties and a great deal of misery so you might as well set up your get-away-from-it-all lounger to work for you.

➤ Choose your equipment wisely. The best recliner or couch for your body has a covering that feels comfortable, with foam or cushioning underneath, and allows some give but still has enough support to help you maintain good postural form.

➤ The armrests should be high enough for you to rest your elbows and forearms without tilting your body from one side to the other to reach them.

➤ The leg and footrests should let your knees bend slightly to allow better circulation in the legs.

➤ That fluffy bedlike pillow looks inviting, but it may be too thick. If it is, it won't allow your head to bend backward into a more relaxed position. Choose a chair with one of these pillows, and you'll simply aggravate and magnify the strain and tension in your mid-back and neck, at the same time that you are becoming aggravated by your favorite basketball team. You can salvage a poorly designed recliner by taking some of the stuffing out of the headrest.

Certainly, one of the biggest pains in the neck occurs when you lean back into an overstuffed cushion that curls your back backward and your head forward. Because your body actually takes this time in the recliner to shape itself and conform to its surroundings, when you get up (with difficulty) from this awkward position, you may have pain. That's why it's crucial to find the support position that properly fits the contours of your back and is comfortable at the same time.

While reclining, open your mouth. It is essential to breathe actively when relaxing. Opening your mouth and breathing in deeply stimulates circulation and oxygen intake. If your body is in a proper position, you won't develop tension in your muscles.

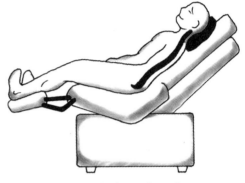

Make the recliner fit YOUR body by unwinding it and extending it backward with support (see Figure 10.4). Did you ever curl up on a terribly uncomfortable couch and swear you'd never do that again? You didn't even feel relaxed, and maybe you even developed some backaches you didn't have before.

Figure 10.4. Reclining during leisure time should also support your body's optimum spinal curves and contours.

Even as you're relaxing lazily in that lounger, take a few moments at regular intervals to flex and extend your feet and clench your fists or relax your hands. When you activate your leg and arm muscles, you'll improve circulation.

Since you are spending some leisure time relaxing, make sure you have clothing that does not inhibit flow or alter your form. Loosen your belt. Take off your shoes; stretch and relax your feet as well.

Footnote in History

Edwin Shoemaker invented the plush, padded rocking and reclining chair that became known as the La-Z-Boy. That familiar name beat out other contest entries such as Sit-N-Snooze, the Slack-Back, and the Comfort Carrier. The first La-Z-Boy lounger was constructed in 1928, but it wasn't until 1961, when television took over America's living rooms, that the comfy lounge chair became a necessity.

THE COUCH POTATO DILEMMA

Most couches and overstuffed chairs tend to be too long in the seat. The distance from the knees to the hips does not allow your back to be positioned into the back cushion very well. When you plop down into a couch like this, you will tend to compensate by lifting one leg up and crossing it over the other to get one knee-space away from the chair edge and be able to sit further back. Some people actually sit cross-legged on the seat.

Perhaps a better way to accommodate a too-long couch or chair is to add a pillow behind your back to decrease the distance between the cushion of the back and the forward edge of the chair or couch. This may, however, be uncomfortable because this type of couch is not designed to provide the best balance or to fit people's forms very well.

If you like to lie on the couch with your head propped up to watch TV, or lie in bed with your head propped up, I must caution you that this activity may cause your body some pain, or worse, which will then carry forward into other aspects of your daily routine.

Getting comfortable and properly balanced in overstuffed furniture may continue to be a challenge until manufacturers of home furniture understand how to be more accommodating to physical form and good balance. That matching sofa and love seat might look terrific in your family room, but they're killing your back. We've made great strides in the office furniture industry. Home furnishings, you're next! For now, I advise you to retrofit the furniture you already have. Use props and pillows to make your furniture conform to you, and be all the wiser when you go furniture shopping.

ARMCHAIR QUARTERBACKING

Carefully consider the position and form of armrests on couches and chairs. If you try to stretch your body or reach an armrest, you end up pulling yourself forward or down and, thus, out of balance. Good balance is not rigid and fixed or uncomfortable.

If the chair doesn't fit, you may also choose to select a different place to sit or recline that serves you better. If you're not in your own home, you may not have many other choices. Best advice: Don't stay long! Even better advice: If you don't want your visitors to stay long, provide extremely uncomfortable chairs!

Dr. Donkin's Shopping Dilemmas

The depth of the couch and firmness of the foam in the seat that you desire are determined by your body size and weight, your thigh, and the length of your lower leg, as well as by your preferred sitting techniques and styles. The density and contour of the backrest also needs to be determined by your sitting form and style (whether you prefer to sit or recline). Also, you have to consider how much time you and others in your household spend on the couch. Whoever logs more "couch time" should get to choose the best initial fit.

My wife and I recently went shopping for a couch for a basement TV room. What a trip! I'm 5'10" and my wife is 5'8". She has long legs and thighs, and I have a long torso. She likes to sit upright and I like to recline. How could we buy a couch we both could benefit from? Here were our choices:

1. I could place a pillow behind my back or behind the cushion I sit in front of because, with my shorter thighs, I need less depth in the couch seat.

2. We could adjust the back cushion to either recline slightly for me or be more upright for my wife.

3. We could buy separate chairs that coordinate but support our individual needs (a couch works for one or both, a separate chair works for one).

What did we do? Our solution was to buy the couch that fit my wife's longer legs, and also buy some fashionable throw pillows so I could fit the couch better, along with our shorter legged children and guests.

KITCHEN TABLE TALK

Where do people seem to gather? Around the kitchen table, of course. But a kitchen (or dining room) chair can be a challenge to sit on for any length of time. If you cannot sit back in the seat and have your back supported properly with the backrest, you can use a small wedge on the seat pan to allow your hips and thighs to be able to tilt forward. You can also use a small amount of fabric to make a little pillow that would fit your back properly. If there is a pillow on the seat pan, you can tilt it forward.

Keep in mind that different family members might have different needs regarding the height and depth of cushions or pillow supports and where to put them. The vertical adjustment of lumbar (lower back) support is critical. If you can't make a chair, such as the kitchen chair, fit you properly, you can achieve support internally by positioning your body properly. Tilt your hips forward so your tailbone guides your lower back into a forward curve, rock your rib cage back, and level your head.

Remember, your children are forming their postures and body habits right now. Help them make good choices that become second nature as they age.

You may not need to spend a great deal of effort, time, or money fitting your kitchen chairs if you use them only once or twice a day, and only for half an hour. Time isn't a big factor in short-term sitting. It's much more important for you to make changes in any automobile seat, recliner, or workplace seating you spend much more of your time using.

If you sit around the kitchen table talking or snacking, you can also just lean back in the chair, prop up your rib cage slightly, and still have a better and more comfortable position than the typical seated slump. Consider changing the height of your kitchen table to encourage better upright balance. (You can saw off the legs, but chances are you might want to go the other way and raise the table with blocks.)

Barstools at kitchen countertops (and in bars) are usually taller than most chairs. Your legs dangle downward, and sometimes the balancing act just to stay perched is challenging. Sit forward on the stool, let your knees drop down so your feet can reach a cross rung on the chair. Better yet, sit on one side of your buttocks and put the opposite foot on the floor. Mom said no elbows on the table, and she's right. But if you must, rest your forearms on the table for balance.

SMART FURNITURE SHOPPING

Looks terrific, matches the carpeting, attractive price, but is it comfortable? Sometimes comfort is the last thing people check when buying furniture. Move comfort up to the top of your list. You're going to spend a lot of time in that chair, couch, or bed, so try this when you shop:

1. Close your eyes after sitting in the chair or couch and put your awareness, in ascending order, into your legs, your back, your chest, then your head, neck, and arms. Can you hold your body in good form and balance?

2. Get in and out of the chair several times. How easy is it?

3. Simulate the tasks and activities you will be performing.

4. Ask someone (preferably a person who is familiar with this book) if you look comfortable, and ask for suggestions if they say you don't.

5. If the cushions in the backrest are too soft or rounded for you, your shoulders will be forced to roll forward and inward in the front, thus accentuating a slumping position. Deep cushy couches may swallow your hips and shoulders, and your hips and legs will tend to roll inward. Pick another style.

HOME/OFFICE COMPUTER

If you spend a significant amount of time—especially if it's intense time—working at a home office or computer for pleasure or work, your computer setup should follow the guidelines for balance, form, and flow discussed throughout this book. Laptops are particularly tricky for good posture because their monitors are low and slumping to look at them becomes the routine position.

AT LEISURE AWAY FROM HOME

Restaurant: Table or booth? Choose whichever suits you, and don't be shy about asking to switch if your initial choice turns out to be uncomfortable. Roll your coat or sweater and put it behind you if the seating needs adjusting.

Stadium Seats/Benches: Can anything be more uncomfortable? Use coats, cushions, and jackets to cushion your buttocks. Angle your knees downward and don't wait for the seventh inning to get up and walk around.

Theater: If you can select your seating, choose the distance that best works for you visually. Some people prefer the back, others the middle. You may even want to wait for cable if you are stuck in the front row during a crowded showing. Instead of craning your neck around the tall guy in front of you, give yourself a little edge by sitting on your rolled-up coat or jacket. If you anticipate problems, take a pillow to sit on or stuff behind you for lower-back support. And a fanny pack can be turned around to fill the space behind your back too.

11. THE ART OF STANDING

Standing seems like the most natural posture. After all, we had to learn to stand before we could walk. Anyone who must stand for a living or who has stood for long periods of time knows that standing can quickly become uncomfortable and tiring. You find yourself looking for the closest wall or post to lean on.

In the standing position, the body is completely vertical, and the same concepts of balance that apply to the upright-seated position also apply to the standing body. Examine your posture and form in the mirror and see how it compares to optimum standing posture.

AN UPHILL BATTLE

What happens frequently with standing, particularly with standing in place, is that the blood must flow from the feet to the heart—uphill. Imagine water trying to flow naturally up Niagara Falls. It can do so only because gravity gets defied with a pump. Likewise, in upright positions, there is a pump in the form of the leg muscles. The body depends on movement of these leg muscles to help squeeze the blood back up through the legs to the heart. Since blood does not move as efficiently uphill against gravity, circulation is affected when the form is not balanced, so you must first make changes in balance when you are standing.

High heels make the pumping task even more difficult because calf muscles are tighter in high heels than in flat shoes. In high heels, your thigh muscles compensate for the imbalance by trying to hold the body in an upright position, but the blood does not flow freely in that position, and fatigue can set in quickly.

When you must stand, either for work or for pleasure, there are things you can do to be comfortable and alert:

➤ Breathe deeply to stimulate your circulation in a standing position.

➤ Tilt your hips and tailbone, and rock the back of your rib cage. This helps you stand for a longer period of time.

➤ Alternately contract and relax your leg muscles.

➤ Your body will naturally seek to move in order to activate the muscles in your arms and legs and stimulate circulation. That's why it is difficult, and not advisable, to stand only in one place for long periods of time.

➤ When standing in one place where you have no choice and can't shift your legs (such as on a crowded subway or bus), you can move your body from side to side, or forward and back, to gain some movement in your body. This isn't as effective as moving your legs and arms, but it is better than not moving at all.

➤ With respect to your body's form, it is advisable to wear clothing that does not interfere with flow, particularly for long stretches of time.

HAZARDOUS DUTY!

If you stand for work, you probably have to assume several positions in the course of a day. Standing jobs generally require reaching, standing in one

---

Roxanne's Story

Roxanne's teenage son became hooked on golf, and she turned into a spectator parent at all the high school tournaments. For her, this meant a great deal of walking and standing around as part of the parental gallery watching the golf events.

The increased standing was taking its toll on Roxanne's lower-back condition. After we talked and I had made her aware of tailbone, rib-cage, and level-head concepts, as well as stretching and stimulating flow, Roxanne was able to watch five matches in six days in four cities without back pain and still remain refreshed. She commented to me that other spectators were complaining of back pain but, for the first time, she wasn't one of them.

place for most of the day, or leaning over a counter or table. Although standing may seem like the easiest part of a job, it can be quite hazardous to your health.

Wear comfortable, low-heeled shoes with a non-slip surface. Many employers specify the type of shoes—even down to color—but make sure they fit properly. If possible, especially if the floor is wet or slippery, request rubber matting to prevent slips and falls. Make sure your shoes have proper arch support and cushioning to absorb the pressure on your upper body from the hard floor surface. In addition, have a small box or step nearby on which you can place one foot. This will ease the pressure on your hips and lower back, as will occasionally alternating your feet on the box.

Keep one or both of your knees bent slightly. The blood flow up the legs depends on your legs' movement, which squeezes the blood up (against gravity) toward the heart. Curl your toes under the ball of your foot and then extend them to improve circulation and decrease stress and strain in the lower legs. Tensing and relaxing your calf muscles also helps.

Keep your body in a natural position. Your spine has a natural curve at the lower back, but when you stand at attention (military style), the curve in your spine is decreased. When you lean forward, the curve also straightens. Try to keep your back in a position that preserves that natural, neutral curve. In addition, minimize twisting. You can vary the curves of your spine by changing the positions of your feet when you are standing. For example, standing with your toes pointed out increases the forward curve of the lower back. "Toeing in" flattens the curve of your lower back.

If you must reach up frequently, for example to remove something or put something on a shelf, use a wide leg stance and position your body so you don't have to twist. Use a stable footstool—one designed for standing. Using unsuitable objects to stand on, such as a chair or a box, increases your chances of an accident. Do use that box, though, for lower shelves. Sit on it while you stock shelves, for example.

Bend at the knees instead of the back. Avoid repeated or prolonged twisting, and stretch your arms, back, legs, and neck before you start.

Standing activities are not limited to the workplace. Your back will be healthier and stronger if you use correct postures at home and play. Brushing teeth, cooking, ironing, sweeping, vacuuming, and other activities that require standing, often in a bent-forward position, can cause problems if you already have back pain, or if your back is fatigued from work.

Checklist for Successful Standing

1. Wear comfortable, low-heeled, non-slip shoes.

2. Use a box as a footrest.

3. Avoid being too rigid.

4. Have everything within easy reach, such as the phone, the register, and the computer.

5. Raise your workstation to prevent your bending forward.

6. Try to change positions, and take stretch breaks frequently.

While performing various standing tasks, it is always a good idea to keep in mind how reaching can affect your balance. For instance, if you are standing at a kitchen counter that is slightly low for your height and form, you will be forced to lean forward. Doing this repeatedly, and over time, can be a factor for your body's form, and if it is, you could bend your knees slightly and spread your feet apart. Regardless, make sure you do counter stretches, with your body in an extended back position, to minimize those undesirable effects.

12. SURVIVE THE DRIVE

Accident prevention should be foremost in your mind when thinking of surviving and thriving. As a driver, you have much power when it comes to preventing accidents. Many factors go into maintaining a safe driving record, not the least of which is your health. Accident prevention starts with a healthy body and mind and continues with avoiding risky situations, such as driving under the influence of alcohol or drugs. Exercise, proper nutrition, and proper breathing are the keys to keeping yourself alert and in control.

WHAT CAUSES ACCIDENTS

Research conducted by the National Highway Traffic Safety Administration (NHTSA) has indicated that the vast majority of traffic accidents in the United States are the result of human error, the three main factors being excessive speed, improper outlook, and inattention. Other factors that cause crashes are brake failure, slick roads, or tire problems.

Excessive speed speaks for itself, but improper outlook includes aggressive driving, driving while under the influence of alcohol or drugs, following too closely, improper lane changes, and running traffic lights. Inattention includes driving while doing other things, like changing radio stations, eating, lighting cigarettes, reaching for objects in the vehicle, talking on cellular phones, and watching pedestrians or other attractions on the side of the road. Inattention also includes fatigue-related symptoms and falling asleep at the wheel.

According to recent studies, 36 percent of fatal accidents were attributed to alcohol (18.2 percent) or excessive speed (18.7 percent). One in every eight crashes resulting in a fatality involves a large truck (over 10,000 lb gross weight), while only 1 percent of the truck drivers involved in the accidents were intoxicated. Although there are more than 7 million large trucks registered in the United States, over the past decade the rate of accidents among these large trucks has declined dramatically; nevertheless, when there is an accident with one of them, it is often deadly.

Whether you drive a large truck or share the road with trucks, you must follow safe driving habits and pay attention. The section immediately following will give you guidelines on how to deal with fatigue while driving. If your body is well-rested, comfortable, and healthy, you will be a safer driver.

FATIGUE

Fatigue is a common complaint. It is often difficult to measure, but is frequently described as a vague tiredness or feeling of low energy, lack of enthusiasm, or weakness. The major causes include all the things we have been talking about: poor posture, bad chair support, and lack of nutrition and exercise.

Counter fatigue by taking breaks or short naps.

IN THE DRIVER'S SEAT

While a lot of attention has been given to office seating, far too little has been given to driver and passenger seating. No matter where you are, your body needs proper individual support, and motor vehicles only create additional challenges.

First, the driver's space is confined on all sides. Second, your legs and feet must control pedals you cannot see. Third, your arms have to reach forward to the steering wheel and controls, and in the meantime, your back is forced into that pain-inducing C-curve.

Not all vehicular body injuries are caused by accidents. The daily insult of riding in a vibrating vehicle can also take a toll on your body, but fortunately there are ways of reducing pressures on it that will result in a more enjoyable ride and a more relaxed state when you reach your destination.

If your car's seats support your posture properly, you will feel better. Incorporate the following guidelines into your driving habits and you should stay more comfortable and alert.

The Basics

➤ Legs—relaxed, not reaching forward;

➤ Feet—flat on the floor or pedal;

➤ Hips—tilted forward;

➤ Torso and Back—square, in balance with good posture;

➤ Arms—relaxed, not reaching forward;

➤ Shoulders—square and over hips; and

➤ Head—straight and looking forward.

INSIDE THE VEHICLE

Seating

For both driver and passenger: First, fit into the seat pan and backrest. Your hips should move into the backrest and the seat pan, with your hips and tailbone tilted forward (see Figure 12.1). The lower back then curves forward over the backrest, with the upper rib cage rocking backward—directly over or behind the hips.

A seat pan that is too long for your thighs will force you to stretch your legs to reach the pedals, or will force you to sit in a poor posture: hips tilting backward and a rounded back. If this is a problem, add a cushion to the backrest.

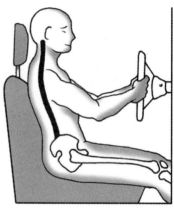

Figure 12.1. The seat, the backrest, the distance the body is from the steering wheel, and the position of the mirrors should all support optimum body postures.

The reach of your legs to the control pedals—the accelerator, the brake, and the clutch—also determines the positioning of your hips and lower back relative to the seat. Keep your feet flat on the floor or pedal. Allow space for some movement.

Backrest

Frequently the backrest of the motor vehicle is slightly reclined because of the smaller space between the floorboard and the roof of the car. The benefit of this is that the weight of your upper body slides into the backrest of the car so your lower back doesn't bear all the weight. Often this reclining position forces your hips to rock backward and your spine to flatten.

Your hips must be tucked underneath the backrest of the seat and your lower spine should be in a curved forward position. It is very important to

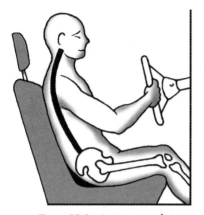

adjust this position to counter the effect of engine vibration and the shock of driving over uneven pavement, potholes, or dips in the road. The vibration from the engine, as well as the movement across uneven or bumpy roads, is basically a form of repetition that will cause fatigue and stress to your body.

If your backrest does not fit properly, allowing a forward tilt of your hips, then retrofit your seat with cushions and wedges to accommodate your physical form (see Figure 12.2). Use cushions, wedges, and padding (even a rolled up towel) to support a balanced position for your form.

Figure 12.2. An improper fit between the seat, the backrest, and the body, as well as poor positioning of the steering wheel and placement of the hands, leads to distorted spinal curves.

Car Seat Materials

Car seats are often made of materials that allow you to sink into them and they do not make for good posture. Although a good marketing ploy because these luxury seats feel so inviting at first, you will come to regret having them, as their lack of support leads to uncomfortable, slumping positions. A good seat in a car should preserve your form and balance, but not be rigid. If the seat is too soft, a lumbar support may help. You can buy one or make one from a rolled towel placed above the buttocks between the lower back and the seat.

Steering Wheel

Your position over the steering wheel can certainly alter the position of your upper body and head, and the distance between your body and your steering wheel is the determining factor for some aspects of your whole body posture. Good body posture also includes neck and shoulder positions, which are often thrust too far forward when driving.

Your arms should be able to comfortably reach the steering wheel. The further you have to reach, the more rounded your shoulders become, causing strain on them and on your neck muscles. Eventually this strained position will cause pain in your shoulders, neck, and back, and will likely give you headaches.

Many times we recommend moving more into the seat or moving the seat closer to the steering wheel, always advising people to make sure they leave enough clearance for the air bag to deploy in the event of a crash.

Headrest

Keep the headrest of your car high enough so that, in the event of an accident, your head does not roll up over the top of it. Set it so the center touches the back of your head at about the height of your ears. Usually, when people begin to use better-balanced positions and postures in motor vehicles, they sit higher in their seats. So move the headrest up (if it is adjustable) to accommodate your new position.

Armrests

Armrests are not easy to change inside a motor vehicle. If you find your arms always resting on something inside the car that is pulling your body away from a balanced and stable position, then don't use the armrests. The armrests inside any motor vehicle should feel comfortable yet provide underlying support for balancing your form.

Rearview Mirror

Adjust the rearview mirror so you have a balanced posture when using the mirror while driving. Take note whether or not you need to adjust your mirror while you are driving. If you need to adjust your mirror downward after you have been driving for a while, that means you are sinking down. Your body posture is being altered adversely, and you should either change your position or get out of the car to take a break and stretch.

Car Ceiling

If you sit upright in your motor vehicle and your head hits the ceiling, then your posture will be altered downward. Keep this is mind when buying an automobile. External safety factors, such as air bags and braking systems, are important, but so are the internal support and safety factors for your body. As Lisa's story demonstrates, the automobile is a challenging environment for initiating change in your body's form.

THE INS AND OUTS OF AUTOMOBILES

Think about how many times you get in and out of a motor vehicle in a week's time. When you're in and out of the car at the cleaners, the grocery, the day-care, the video store, and finally back home, you could even feel as though you had just done a stretch of aerobic exercise. But if you adjust your car seat properly and learn the ins and outs of getting in and out, you will use repetition to enhance your balance and form just while doing your daily chores.

Getting into a Car: Aim your tailbone for the spot where the back of the seat meets the backrest. Then rotate your shoulders and hips at the same time by pulling on the steering wheel to position yourself.

Getting out of a Car: Rotate your hips and shoulders together. Step out and grab the doorframe, steering wheel, or car seat to help push yourself out. Just after exiting the car, do some back extensions to improve the flow in your body.

Lisa's Story

Lisa traded cars with her brother. His was newer, more reliable for her long commute to work, and got better gas mileage. But no one anticipated the wear and tear the "new" car would have on Lisa.

The steering wheel in this car was more difficult to turn than in her previous car, so she had adopted the habit of turning the steering wheel with only her dominant right hand, thereby overusing it. Because she sat lower and further away from the steering wheel, her problems got even more complicated since, from this leverage point, she strained her right forearm and shoulder every time she turned the wheel.

The added strain began to show up as pain in her shoulder and right arm. I suggested to Lisa that she adjust the seat with props, such as pillows, to raise her higher and closer to the steering wheel. She took my advice and is now driving happily without strain.

New cars might be alluring, but if you can't adjust them to fit your form (even in the short-term with a rental car or loaner), they're not a smart choice for you after all.

Getting into a Tall Vehicle: (a truck or sports utility vehicle): Step up with your left foot (if you're driving) and slide your right foot and leg under the steering wheel. Then follow the same procedure you would in a car. Rotate your shoulders and hips at the same time, and make sure you are sitting with your tailbone and hips deep in the seat and backrest.

Getting out of a Tall Vehicle: Rotate your hips and shoulders together. Step down with your left foot and slide out while using the doorframe or steering wheel for balance. NEVER jump out of a vehicle.

ASSISTING SMALL CHILDREN

Lifting children in and out of car seats and safety restraints is almost an aerobic exercise in itself. Parents, grandparents, and other caregivers perform this task as a natural part of driving, yet the techniques are often overlooked. First, consider how many times you lift a child in and out of a car safety seat. Is it every day, week after week, month after month? If it is, then it is a good idea to check out your vehicle—without any children around.

First, secure the safety seat according to the manufacturer's instructions. In recent traffic surveys, it was found that many people did not have the car seats secured safely. If you have questions, contact the manufacturer through their toll-free number or website. Your local safety council or police department can also provide information.

Once the seat is safely secured in the backseat, practice your moves so you can decide ahead of time the best and easiest procedure for you.

➤ Place your knee on the vehicle's seat to support you closer to the child seat. Keep good body balance and don't overreach.

➤ Try to get the child to help (if the child is old enough to lift his or her arms and crawl into the seat).

➤ A struggling, screaming child can often put you into awkward body positions. Simply stop and start over. Do your best to calm the child.

➤ You may want to stretch and breathe before or after you lean into the vehicle (afterward might be easier because the child is safely secured).

➤ Take your car seat along when you're vehicle shopping. See how easy or difficult it is to get kids in and out of it. That may be the deciding factor in your purchase decision.

TRAVEL TIPS

Take your wallet and any other bulky items out of your pockets before getting into the car, especially for long-distance trips. Bulky items press against your hip and thigh and can cause pinched nerves and reduced blood circulation to the legs, resulting in pain, numbness, and weakness.

Take a five-minute break for every hour on the road. During that break, get out of the car, stretch, close your eyes and allow them to relax and focus on something other than the road. Do the Sixty-Second Stand-Up, Perk-Up Break. (See Chapter 10.)

Time will take its toll, whether you're taking frequent trips around town running errands, commuting to and from work, shuttling children, or taking longer trips on vacation. Use repetition to make a positive imprint on your balance and form. Stretch and move to keep flow stimulated. Smile. You are accomplishing great things for your body for a long time to come.

LIFTING OUT OF A CAR TRUNK

Everyone has occasion to lift something out of a car trunk. When you have to unload something, a lawn mower, the groceries, lumber for a renovation, or all the odds and ends in your car's trunk, here's how to do it safely:

1. Place your foot on the bumper, or in the trunk;
2. Maintain your proper spinal curves;
3. Put your hand or elbow on the car for support;
4. Pull the load as close as possible;
5. Place the load on the edge of the trunk for leverage;
6. Position yourself as close to the load as possible;
7. Press your legs against the car;
8. Bend from the hips with your back slightly arched;
9. Get a good grip and test the load;
10. Make sure the load is pulled up as close as possible;
11. Head up, lift the load smoothly while bracing;
12. Place the load close to the body for normal carrying;
13. Carry the load safely to its destination.

13. Activities

HOUSEWORK

Most accidents happen at home, primarily, of course, because you're home a lot and you are doing everyday tasks that involve stretching, bending, reaching, and kneeling. It's always the activity you least expect that may cause you pain the next day (if not immediately). Remember what you know about alignment, balance, form, and flow, and let these principles be your guide to daily activities.

Take household tasks, for example. How often do you reach to the very top of the linen closet for that blanket? Once, twice a year? Or climb a ladder and reach to sink a nail into the siding of your house? Not too often. These occasional, unfamiliar activities, if not done properly (with step stools and care), can cause strain and pain.

Using the principles of balance and form are even more important when performing everyday chores, such as scrubbing the floor, sweeping, and vacuuming. Pay attention to the contortions you're putting your body into and use the examples in this book to devise better ways of accomplishing your tasks. You can always delegate them to your teenager (if there's one around), but seriously, doing chores around the house is a very good way to put movement into your day—and is just as vital as a walk around the block or a spin on a bicycle. Michio Kushi, the Macro-biotic guru, offers housework as the organic way of getting effective daily exercise.

AROUND THE HOUSE

Before performing any unaccustomed physical activities, it's a good idea

Jody's Story

Jody winced her way into my office and erupted in tears after she entered the treatment room. Just a week before, she had remarked on how good she was feeling and how the new exercise plan I had recommended had helped her to sleep, and had improved her stamina during hectic workdays.

This day was different, however. Instead of an alarm clock, a sharp, piercing pain, extending from the right side of her neck to the right shoulder, awakened her. The pain and accompanying muscles spasms clearly indicated that something had happened, but she could not recall anything she'd done that might have resulted in an injury.

As we began looking back at her activities for the previous week, she recalled how she had been pruning some shrubs the day before. She described using a long-handled pruning shear and demonstrated her technique: holding her arms out to the side, almost parallel to the ground, to get enough leverage to cut the thick branches. To see these branches, she had held her head in a forced, flexed position. Although Jody only pruned for an hour, she admitted to working at a feverish pace so she could get ready to go out that night.

I explained that holding her arms extended, with her elbows far away from her body, while forcing her head downward, concentrated forces and strain into the exact area of the pain she was experiencing. She had her head turned to the right most of the time, she said, which explained why the pain was greater on that side. Having explained the origins of this problem to her, I went on to give her the proper positions to assume when pruning or performing similar tasks. After her pain cleared up, she took my recommendations and is now pruning happily and safely, with no return of her former, excruciating, pain.

to prepare your body by figuring out which areas of it you are going to use, and then stretching them. Stretch during and after these activities as well, to insure proper flow. And pace yourself. You will lessen the risk of strain if you go at unaccustomed activities less intensely—no matter how much of a hurry you're in—and take it easy on your muscle groups. If not, those muscles will remind you tomorrow that you haven't.

Vacuuming is seldom the most pleasant household chore, and it can be even more unpleasant if it causes muscle strain and gnawing irritation every time you do it. Before you give up and replace all your carpet with tile, however, consider the proper way to vacuum. Prepare for it by stretching to improve flow. Try a few simple warm-ups with back, shoulder, and neck stretches. And while you are vacuuming, stop occasionally to take some deep breaths.

The best way to become aware of how vacuuming or other household activities affect the body is to look at someone else doing these things. Or take a glance at yourself in the mirror. Are you stooping forward so your posture is off-balance? Do you twist your upper body and shoulders, concentrating all the force in your shoulders while you push and pull?

Once you see yourself, or someone else, vacuuming incorrectly (never mind the corners!), try again. Only this time, distribute the force and leverage of your pushing and pulling by stepping forward and back with your legs. Don't overreach with your arms and shoulders. You'll find this technique is actually easier. You might also bend your knees slightly and hold your body in a more upright and balanced position. Periodically push on your thigh with your free hand to gain some extra leverage.

Whether you use an upright vacuum or a canister-type with a nozzle, you'll want to put the handle in the best position to accommodate your

Doug's Story

Doug walked ahead of me from the exam room to the x-ray room. Normally over six feet tall, his severe back pain and accompanying muscle spasms had reduced him to 5 feet 7 inches, and he walked sideways and tilted forward.

Doug knew a severe back injury when he felt it, and after he had slipped and fallen in an abrupt twisting motion that morning, he had immediately applied ice packs and called me. His pain was difficult enough, but added to this was his disappointment because he had been planning to take part in a bicycle race in seven weeks.

He made a strong improvement, but against his better judgment and my recommendations, he admitted that he had taken a bike ride less than a week after the injury. He did do back and leg stretches before he rode, he said, and when his back began to hurt after a few minutes' ride, he stopped and lowered the seat. This served to bow his back inward and keep his head up, and he reported that it made him feel much better, as did the exercises beforehand, and he was able to continue his bike riding. His conscientious exercise and stretching efforts, combined with his attention to good riding postures, enabled him to compete and finish the race without further injury.

height. If you're shorter, you can increase your leverage by holding the handle lower.

Taking your bike out for a spin can be demanding on your arms, shoulders, and neck, so do some preparatory stretches. And while you are out riding, alternately redistribute the weight and position of your arms, hands, and wrists on the handlebars and grips, and lower the seat. You'll sit taller and much more comfortably for your back.

LIFTING

Whether it's groceries, files, car parts, cartons, containers, cases, luggage, or whatever else we lift during the course of our day at home or at work, it is important to know how to lift properly.

Proper Lift

1. Adopt a broad-based or diagonal stance;

2. Maintain spinal curves;

3. Move the load close;

4. Use the legs;

5. Squat lower for deeper lifts;

6. Keep the head up;

7. Now lift.

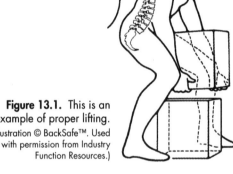
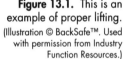

Figure 13.1. This is an example of proper lifting. (Illustration © BackSafe™. Used with permission from Industry Function Resources.)

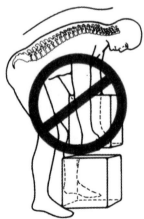

Improper Lift

1. Spinal curves not maintained;

2. Resulting posture forces the body to use the spinal ligaments;

3. The load is too far away;

4. The position is prone to injury;

Figure 13.2. This is an example of improper lifting. (Illustration © BackSafe™. Used with permission from Industry Function Resources.)

5. The deeper lifts in this position also increase the potential for injury (see a healthcare professional for help).

Support belts should never be used as a substitute for a proper lifting technique. Support belts tend to make people believe they can lift heavier loads (weighing 25 percent more) than they can without a belt. The excessive use of these belts for lifting will, in fact, make the supporting lower back and abdominal muscles weak, and will make you more prone to injury. Belts are useful for occasional heavy exertion and unaccustomed tasks (like moving your piano), but that is all.

14. TO REST, TO SLEEP, PERCHANCE TO BE COMFORTABLE

FATIGUE AND REST IN TRUCKS AND HUMANS

Perpetual motion might be a phenomenon in physics and other sciences that deal with the universe at a molecular level. However, perpetual motion for a truck could have deadly consequences. Trucks need rest, just as humans do. Without cool-down or warm-up periods, mechanical efficiency is compromised and breakdown or horrific accidents can follow.

Rest periods for trucks allow systems to cool down, and also allow time for inspection and repair. If a truck were to run non-stop as inevitable minor problems occurred, those minor problems would soon develop into major problems. Oil leaks, cracks in belts, worn brakes, and other small defects would become major, life-endangering problems.

Warm-up periods are also important in proper truck management. For example, on a bitterly cold day with a wind-chill factor of –30°F, fluids in the truck would be too thick to function properly, and braking systems, fuel systems, and lubrication systems would be compromised. No matter what the temperature is, it's good truck-handling to include a warm-up period in the pre-trip checklist. Appropriate warm-up and cool-down periods extend the longevity of the truck and decrease the risk of accident and personal injury.

As with trucks, your body needs periods of proper rest and sleep, free of disorders, as it uses those periods to counteract the stresses and strains of your day. Sleep disorders, restless or fitful sleeping habits, or poor sleeping postures can contribute to, or aggravate, many physical conditions, such as degenerative arthritis, fibrositis, muscle and ligament strain, or spinal misalignment (see Figure 14.1). Since all these factors may directly or indirectly contribute to backaches, headaches, neck aches, or any other

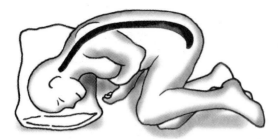

Figure 14.1. Sleeping in a curled position causes a less optimum spinal position.

pains you may experience during your waking hours, it is imperative that you rest and sleep well.

And proper sleeping positions are important for the quality rest you need. When you are sitting upright, the forces of gravity are pulling down on the bones and discs of your spine, and the muscles and ligaments are hard at work supporting you in a vertical position. During sleep, however, you are horizontal, gravity is no longer compressing the length of your body, and your muscles and ligaments can relax. You must, however, sleep in a good position to reap the full benefits of a good night's sleep.

As we will discuss further in this chapter, the two most beneficial sleeping positions are on your back or on your side. Stomach sleeping forces your spine and neck to twist, which does not give the muscles and ligaments in those areas the rest and rejuvenation that sleep is intended to. In fact, this unnatural twisting compounds muscle and ligament strain and spinal misalignment. You can effectively reduce or eliminate the negative forces of gravity on your spine, muscles, and ligaments by adopting sleeping positions that are the most beneficial for your body. Using properly supportive bedding, as we will discuss further on, is also important.

Sleep cycles are another consideration when setting yourself up for a good night's sleep. Before falling asleep, a period of drowsiness occurs, brought on by a lowering of your body temperature. Then comes sleep. The normal sleep cycle lasts about ninety minutes, and includes several periods of light sleep that gradually lead to very deep sleep, and then back again to light sleep, before the cycle starts anew.

By getting up at the same time every morning, even on weekends and holidays, you reset your body clock and recycle all your sleep and wake cycles to your benefit. Waking up late one day may throw off your next day's cycles.

Be cautious about using drugs to help you sleep. Sleep-inducing drugs should be used under careful supervision and only in special cases. Using them on your own for long periods of time may allow any drug residues in your body to carry over into the daytime and cause dull thinking as well as slow reflexes. Alcohol-induced sleep is also of poor quality because, as a depressant, alcohol minimizes deep sleeping and causes you to wake frequently. Nicotine, too, interferes with quality sleep because it is a central nervous system stimulant. And the caffeine found in sodas, chocolate, and many common pain relievers can have stimulating effects that last at least six hours.

MAKING SLEEP WORK FOR YOU

Set the proper stage for sleep, and you can make it work for you, not against you (see Figure 14.2). The quality of your sleep has a major impact on the quality of your life. Sleep not only helps to counteract the everyday physical and mental assaults on your body, it also charges your battery and rejuvenates you so you can participate in each day's activities with enthusiasm and positive expectations. If you wake up rested and refreshed, it's easier to start the day with a positive attitude.

During an average week, you spend about as much time sleeping as you do working, so it's important to make the most of those sleeping hours. In order to get the most out of your sleep and face the day with maximum energy, you may need to change some of your customary sleeping habits.

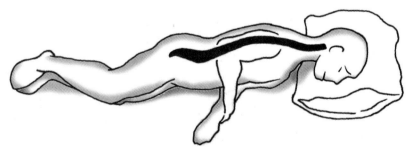

Figure 14.2. The natural flow of spinal curves should be intact during sleep.

ABOUT BEDDING

The sleeping surface of both the mattress and the pillows should fit your form to give your body a good balance while in this reclining position. Although gravity is not as much a factor in the sleeping position as it is when sitting or standing upright, it still subtly affects how you fit into your bedding surface. Gravity will pull your body downward, and the support you have in your bedding and pillow should respect that downward pull and fit your form. The goal is to make the core of your body, from your neck to your hips, parallel with the floor.

When purchasing a bedding set, you should make sure it is large enough and firm enough for your comfort. Test the mattress by lying down on it for a full five minutes, with your partner if you share a bed, and don't be intimidated by the store surroundings. Your comfort is what matters.

As you lie down to sleep at night, you relieve the forces of gravity that have been compressing your body all day. The bedding you choose must be able to support the weight of your body without sagging, and yet be pliable enough to accommodate the contours of your spine, hips, shoulders, neck, and head.

Bedding that sags places extra strain on your body when you are supposed to be relaxed and supported, and you may end up carrying that strain into the next day's activities. So, replace or repair your faulty bedding when necessary. The Better Sleep Council recommends replacing a mattress every eight to ten years. If you are unsure what type of bedding would work best for you, consult a doctor of chiropractic who has a thorough understanding of your body mechanics.

If you have certain gastrointestinal, respiratory, or sinus conditions that require you to sleep propped up instead of fully horizontal, the bedding and pillow surfaces should still be able to accommodate your form.

THE MATTRESS GAME

The right bedding for you is largely a personal decision. Some people prefer a very firm bedding surface, while others like a soft pillow feel to their mattress. Regardless, there are basic guidelines for ensuring a better night's sleep. Of course, as in all other aspects of your environment, your bed should support your form and encourage flow.

If you awake in the night or morning with back, hip, neck, or shoulder pains, that is a sign of an ill-fitting sleeping surface or a poor sleeping technique.

Conventional mattresses with box springs tend to be most people's sleeping surface of choice. And, just like people, mattresses come in a variety of sizes and shapes. If your mattress is too hard (and many futons are very hard), you risk injury to pressure points, which may evolve into irritations and other painful conditions over time. If that's the case, you can place quilted fiber or foam mattress pads on top of your mattress to achieve some measure of comfort and still benefit from the underlying support.

If your mattress is too soft (the Goldilocks dilemma), then your body will bend, twist, and deform to a hammock position. Deforming to conform can be OK for a short period of time (a weekend at your mother-in-law's), but you will create misery for yourself if this practice continues over your sleeping and waking lifetime.

Airbeds have become increasingly popular. In addition to being handy, they have several intriguing benefits. You can custom fit an airbed to fit you by adjusting the firmness, and the leg, hip, and upper-back controls. The larger airbeds even have dual controls so each person can adjust to his or her side.

Water beds now come in a variety of wave forms and densities. If you have to struggle to get in and out of your water bed, that's not good. Heated water beds can be soothing for muscle tension and soreness. And if you suffer from any joint conditions, such as arthritis, the floating feel of water can be quite comfortable, while the gentle movement caused by your breathing can actually stimulate flow.

Hotel beds can be murder on your back and neck because most beds and pillows are too soft. People equate comfort with fluffiness, but it's support that ends up being more comfortable over time—and healthier. Try asking for a king-size bed next time because kings are usually firmer. And try to sleep diagonally across the bed to avoid the dip in an often-used mattress. Check out the beds before you check in!

PILLOW FIGHT

The contour of your pillow should be designed to fill the space between your neck and your head in the bed so that your head is comfortably supported in a good position (see Figure 14.3).

Now the question is: What type of pillow should I use? The answer is: Whichever pillow allows you to fall asleep and stay asleep. Here are some choices:

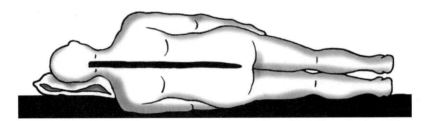

Figure 14.3. Your mattress and pillow should allow for the contours of your body to be supported so that the spine is parallel to the floor and the hips and shoulders are perpendicular to the floor.

➤ Pillows filled with buckwheat hulls can give a custom fit, but they tend to be noisy and can feel too hard for many people.

➤ Feather pillows are soft in texture but usually compress too easily and do not support form.

➤ Regular fiber-filled pillows vary in their compression but can be bunched up to side sleep, or stretched out for back sleeping.

➤ Memory foam contour pillows can give a good fit for backside sleeping, but may compress too much when sleeping on the side, especially as the pillow ages. (Memory foam compresses when you apply pressure but resumes its original form when the pressure is removed.)

➤ Fluid-filled pillows offer unique fitting for the head, neck, and shoulder contours, but are heavier and can leak.

➤ Check out your options before you buy, if possible.

POSTURE YOURSELF FOR SLEEP

The two best sleeping positions, as we said, are on your back or on your side. Once you are in bed, prepare yourself for sleep: stretch lengthwise, reaching your arms above your head, and pointing your toes toward the foot of the bed. This helps relax you and prepare you for assuming a comfortable and correct sleeping position, the best-balanced position (open, not curled-up) that also encourages flow. As you are falling asleep, try to make your breathing deeper and more rhythmic.

Some tossing and turning is normal as you sleep. But with the help of supportive bedding and a good pillow, combined with the proper sleeping postures, your nights are sure to be more restful.

Of course, during periods of sleep, you are not consciously aware of your posture and your form. But you do have conscious control over your body's position when you initiate sleep, and this can, over time, carry over into better sleeping positions for the duration of your time asleep. If your sleeping position is awkward, it could be that your body is compensating for conditions and habits you've acquired in your waking daily routine. It can serve as a clue to examine other areas of your routine to make any needed changes and improvements.

BACK SLEEPERS

Back sleepers will want to make sure they use their pillow to reinforce their neck's forward curve (see Figure 14.4). A thin pillow is usually best because it can be shaped to curl under your neck and support its natural forward curve. Specially designed contour pillows are available and they may cost more, but the price is worth it if you find one that fits your body and sleeping style.

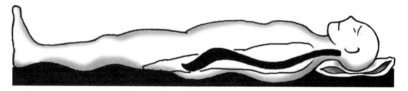

Figure 14.4. Your mattress and pillow should allow support for your body contours so that your spinal curves are intact.

Another consideration for back sleepers: Avoid sleeping with your arms above your head. This puts a strain on your shoulders and upper arms, and can crowd your neck vertebrae. A common symptom is numbness in your arms and hands. Some say you should never sleep with your arms anywhere but at your side.

If you find you must sleep on two or three pillows when lying on your back, then your form has undoubtedly been altered enough that your mid-back is curved quite prominently forward. As you are making changes in other areas, you may carefully, and gradually, make key changes in your body's flexibility by stretching and fitting better into your sleeping environment. A better fit means adopting a more open position on your side with your knees bent, and a better sleeping environment refers to using a pillow that supports your neck and head, and a mattress that supports the curves of your body. You can start sleeping on a thinner pillow, but, in most cases, you should not do this without the advice of your healthcare provider.

SIDE SLEEPERS

For side sleepers, there are also a few tricks. Your pillow should fill the space between your neck and the bed, so that your neck is level with the bed. Keeping in mind that your spine should be parallel to the floor is another way to monitor your sleeping position. This position keeps your neck, head, and shoulder from crowding and jamming the vertebrae on the side of your neck that is closest to the bed. It also keeps the opposite side of your neck from stretching. As we said, a specially designed pillow can come to the rescue because it will keep your neck parallel to the bed's surface.

Again, avoid sleeping with your arm jammed up under your neck and head as it can result in numbness in your arms and hands. Try to tuck the shoulder closest to the bed slightly forward, with your forearm across your stomach or lying on the bed. Remember not to tuck your chin (see Figure 14.5). Keep your head up, with your face parallel to the bed.

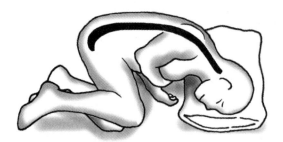

Figure 14.5. Sleeping on your side in a curled position pulls your body out of balance.

Side sleepers should keep their legs on top of each other with knees bent. If you throw your top leg over toward the bed, it makes your hips twist and rotates your pelvis and lower spine. Keep your knees together or place the upper knee slightly behind the lower one. A thin pillow between your knees helps maintain this position.

The tendency to curl up into a ball is very common. It's not detrimental to do this occasionally, but adopting it as your primary sleeping position is not desirable because it pulls your body out of balance and accentuates poor form.

I rarely recommend sleeping on your stomach, yet many people do. It twists your lower back, neck, and head in awkward ways, but if you must do it, you can sleep angled slightly forward from the side, as long as you keep in mind that your form *should* be in a more balanced position.

Consider the room temperature in order to stimulate flow by getting your body as warm as you like it to be. The clothes you sleep in should not inhibit the flow of blood in your body and should not inhibit your body's ability to breathe in deeply and regularly.

If you prop yourself up in bed to read, make sure the pillows create a balance for your form.

THE RIGHT SIDE OF GETTING OUT OF BED

How to get out of bed is important too.

1. Lie on your side facing the direction in which you plan to get out of bed.

2. Place your legs close to the edge but not dangling.

3. Use the top arm to push yourself up to a sitting position.

4. As you begin to assume a seated position, use your bottom arm, the one closest to the bed's surface, to provide additional support as you rise.

5. At the same time, let your legs slip out of bed and let your feet drop to the floor as you sit up.

6. After you get up, do some stretches, such as back extensions, side stretches, and arm, leg, and shoulder stretches.

Keep a record of your sleeping habits for twenty-one days and watch how your conscious thought and action can result in new sleeping habits that become second nature. Don't be discouraged if it takes some time and effort. The reward of waking up refreshed each day is well worth it.

Sleep habits that include good posture, personalized sleep schedules, and the elimination of alcohol, caffeine, drugs, and nicotine will revitalize you and allow you to start fresh each day. A good night's sleep will make you more alert and will reduce the risk of fatigue-related injury.

15. A BETTER WAY TO WALK FOR HEALTH

Nearly all of us walk every day, if only to get around the house, to the car, and to the office. But are we doing it right and are we getting all the benefits of walking?

THE OBVIOUS BENEFITS OF WALKING

➤ Walking is an excellent choice of EXERCISE.

➤ Walking is EASY. You already know how to do it.

➤ Walking is SAFE, especially if you warm up first, know when to stop, and have a safe walking route.

➤ Walking is CHEAP. You only need a good pair of walking shoes.

➤ And, walking can be done almost anywhere, in any weather, and at any time—with just a few precautions. A mere thirty minutes of walking a day will be extremely beneficial for your health!

WALKING WITH STYLE

As you begin walking for health, remember that a correct walking posture reduces the chance of injury. Begin by walking slowly for about five minutes to warm up your muscles, and then gradually speed up. Walk with your head and chin up and your shoulders back. Try to hold your stomach in. Keep your back upright, but not rigid. Keep the curves of your spine as natural as possible. Don't lean forward.

As you walk, lift your feet up so they come completely off the pavement. Land on your heel and roll forward to push off again with your toes.

Keep your toes pointed straightforward, let your arms swing naturally, and breathe fully!

Walk at a comfortable pace. Your pace will change as you become used to walking. Pace yourself so you can hold a conversation with another person without gasping for air.

THE RIGHT EQUIPMENT
Shoes

There are many different types of walking shoes. The kind you need depends on the intensity of your walk and the surface on which you walk. Your shoes should be comfortable and should support your whole foot. A reputable athletic shoe store can guide you. Be sure you are standing while they measure BOTH feet.

Clothing

Clothing must NOT constrict your body movements. In very hot weather, clothing made of fabric that breathes can help keep you cool. In cooler weather, wear layers that can be removed as you warm up. In freezing weather or snow, walk indoors. Cold muscles and slippery ice increase your risk of injury.

Belongings

Carry as light a load as possible. If you must carry keys, money, or other small items, use a hip or backpack. Carrying a shoulder bag may throw your body off balance.

Ankle and Wrist Weights

Though some studies have found that wearing wrist weights can burn calories more quickly, they are not generally a good idea for beginners.

Ankle weights place too much pressure on the knees and back.

WALK YOUR WALK

Walk so you are comfortable, keeping your physical condition in mind. Make sure you feel good about the way you are walking and bear in mind the following:

➤ Your stride should be equal for each leg. Beginners should use a shorter stride and concentrate more on posture. More experienced walkers use a medium stride. A long stride provides the greatest stretch and is generally used by experienced and competitive walkers.

➤ Change your rhythm occasionally. Listen to music, if it's safe, on a track or trail where there is no vehicular traffic, and do not have the volume so high you can't hear what's behind you. You should always be aware of your surroundings and keep safety foremost in your mind.

➤ Let your arms swing naturally. Speed walkers may want to bend their arms at a ninety-degree angle and pump them because this adds force to the walk.

➤ Keep your posture in check. Your posture is affected by the position of your spine, your head, and your eyes. Keep the natural curves of your spine without being rigid. Keep your head up and look straight ahead. But make sure, too, that you are aware of the surface you are walking on so you do not trip or step in a hole or off a curb.

➤ Cool down. When you return from your walk, take about five minutes to stretch and shake out your muscles.

If you ever experience pain while walking, STOP! See your healthcare provider and describe your symptoms and what you were doing at the time. He or she may be able to customize a walking program to relieve your pain.

LEARNING NEW HABITS

Habits are learned responses acquired over time. Consequently, it may take several weeks for you to add walking as a positive new habit. You may have to convert old habits into new ones, correct ones. Observe your actions and note the failures and the improvements. Allow yourself to make corrections without scolding yourself. Give yourself a pat on the back when you see improvements. And don't be discouraged if it takes some time and effort. The benefits of walking regularly are well worth it!

16. FREQUENT FLYER CARRY-ONS AND CARRY-ABOUTS

If one size fits all, then airline seats really don't fit anybody. First-class airline seats can be fairly comfortable because they recline farther and the leg rests raise higher than other seats. But when it comes to most of us who travel in business or coach, the seats can be a downright pain in the back.

Even an hour in a compromising position can put you at risk for pain. And pain is not in your business or leisure travel plans so, until airlines sit up and take notice, try these tips:

➤ Use pillows and blankets to support your neck and back.

➤ If the headrest is movable, adjust it to fit your head; if you're tall, move it up.

➤ Use the leg and foot rests, if any, to change position more often. The larger seats in business class allow you to use blankets and pillows (found in the overhead bins) to fill in where you need padding. You can use these in coach too; it's just a little tighter.

➤ Coach seats don't usually fit the natural contours of any body. The flared sides provide lateral support, but they aren't much help to people who are too big or too small for the seat.

➤ Book an aisle seat and stick your legs out into the aisle when food carts and people aren't moving past.

➤ Wear loose-fitting, comfortable clothing.

➤ Keep your shoes on (wear comfortable shoes, such as athletic shoes). Cabin pressure may cause your feet to swell.

➤ Remove your wallet and any other bulky objects from your hip pockets.

➤ Place your books or laptops on the fold-down tray table, or in your lap on top of pillows. Be aware, though, that anything in your lap tends to make your neck flex forward awkwardly. Bend your elbows at a ninety-degree angle.

➤ Exercise. Follow the simple examples in this chapter.

HOW TO CARRY ON

Obviously, you don't want to drag all your worldly possessions through O'Hare Airport. Nor do you want to risk hurting your back by running for a flight while dragging a briefcase, carry-on bag, purse, coat, magazine, and coffee. Travel light and travel smart. Balance what you're carrying to keep your spine aligned.

People carry all kinds of things: book bags, beepers, briefcases, cell phones, laptops, and purses that they must transport while walking. (There are now regulations in U.S. airports that limit carry-ons to two pieces, and they could actually do your back a favor). When carried improperly, these items may alter your body balance. If, for instance, you carry a purse on one side most of the time, your body will shift in several possible ways to accommodate for the extra load on that one side. Add to your imbalance a pair of ill-fitting or structurally unsound shoes, or high heels, and you can do some serious damage to your body.

If you are carrying a purse over your shoulder, observe the space between your body and your arm so you can get an idea of how the purse should hang to fit your form. If the purse or other item is slung too low, it can cause your body to shift to one side, or cause your shoulder to drop or rise. You can also try moving your arm outward about ten degrees from the side of your body to gain a little more space for items you may be carrying. More than ten degrees might cause extra muscle activity and strain in your shoulders and neck.

Straps of purses and other shoulder-bearing items should be wider, with some padding to distribute the weight. They should fit the contour of the space between your neck and shoulder and be angled so the straps do not dig into your shoulder muscle itself. Narrow straps in this area can actually cause a reduction in flow through the muscles and can alter the function and movement of some of your neck and shoulder muscles.

To carry a purse with a long strap comfortably, put the strap over your head and settle the strap on your left or right shoulder and across your body diagonally so the purse is under the right or left arm. This is a simple solution, and a safe one in high-crime areas or when traveling because the bag won't slip off your shoulder or be easily taken from you.

Depending on how you walk with side-carrying items, such as a brief-case or a laptop, you may tend to tip forward or backward. Luggage carts and bags with wheels will also tend to pull you to one side.

MOVING ABOUT WITH BACKPACKS AND BOOK BAGS IN BALANCE

The way most people carry backpacks and book-bag-type bags is with one strap over one shoulder (see Figure 16.1). This creates an off-balance position. The contents are usually heavy too. It would be better to use both straps—one over each shoulder as the pack was designed to be carried— even though it might be a little awkward getting it on and off. Also, if the book bag is carried too low or too high, it can cause you to bend forward too far to stay balanced in an upright position. You should adjust the straps so the bag fits into the hollow of your back. Over time and with repetition, this would have a cumulative beneficial effect.

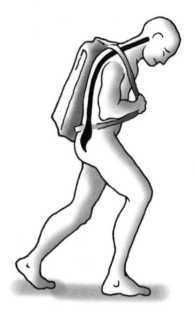

Figure 16.1. Improper distribution of books and materials in a book bag, combined with improper carrying, can lead to continued poor postures, as well as back pain and muscle tension.

Many times, with backpacks for instance, you will shift or twist your body to get out of a car's seat, carrying the backpack at the same time. This wrenching position is aggravating to the back, neck, shoulders, and legs. Instead, place the bag in the car before you get in and conversely, get out of the car before retrieving the bag. Use the proper lifting techniques.

Take a look in the mirror without any of the items you normally carry. Look at your posture from the front and from the side, and use a mirror to

Tracy's Story

Tracy was ready to pull her hair out if she could have just grasped it firmly. She had trouble holding anything in her right hand. What had started out as an ache in her forearm and a pain in her shoulder had progressed into a numbness and tingling, and a weakness in her right wrist and hand. In general, her entire right arm ached.

Doctors had prescribed a variety of medications, but nothing had worked. When I first saw Tracy for this problem, I saw classic signs of carpal tunnel syndrome, but as we assessed her typical daily routine, I realized there was more to her discomfort.

Her symptoms and conditions were cumulative. She had difficulty sleeping because she slept in a curled-up side position, with a pillow that was not thick enough to support her neck, so her head was scrunched to the right, and her right shoulder was jammed upward toward her ear. Her arms were folded under her head, wrists flexed inward, and hands clenched together.

When she finally mustered enough energy to get out of bed, she rode an exercise bike for fifteen minutes to help her body wake up. As she showed me how she positioned her body on the bike, I observed that her wrists were in a sideways tilted position on the handlebars, which added to the strain on her wrists and forearm. She also held her head straight down, occasionally closed her eyes, and lowered her back, thereby putting herself in the exact opposite of a good balanced position for bike riding.

I examined how she routinely carried her purse. Although her purse was moderately sized, it felt as though she were carrying a ton of bricks in it. She, of course, carried it over her ailing right shoulder, and, adding insult to injury (literally), she rested her forearm and hand on the purse when she was walking. This naturally caused the strap to dig even deeper into the muscle between her neck and shoulder.

At work as a travel agent, Tracy wore a headset because she was on the phone constantly. That's the good news. But she sat on the edge of her seat, in a forward slump position, to look at a computer monitor that was too low. Her keyboard was too high, and she used a mouse that was positioned too far to the right.

look over your shoulder at your body balance from the back. Now grab your purse or your briefcase—whichever you normally carry. Observe how your balance is changed. Once you are able to see how your balance shifts, you can make subtle changes in the length of the straps, or in the way you carry items, so you can bring your balance more toward a center position.

No wonder she was in pain. Let's unravel Tracy's condition and let me also give you the specific instructions that allowed her to take control of her environment and make changes to aid her body balance, form, and flow.

- When she slept, Tracy added a pillow that fit and was comfortable. By easing the strain on her neck, she was able to sleep in a more open position, and she learned to relax her arms and hands when she initiated sleep. She also took my advice to try some deep breathing and slow stretching exercises before she went to bed.

- On her exercise bike, she modified the handlebars to add more padding and to be softer, and changed the position of her hands and wrists on them. I helped her discover a better-balanced, full-body posture for the bike, and suggested she adjust her seat to accommodate this position. Early morning stretches for the arms and shoulders took about a minute and were helpful as she began her day.

- Guess what was in that purse—at least nine dollars in pennies, nickels, dimes, and quarters. She also removed other things that weren't essential, but added weight. When she was ready to shop for another purse, she looked for a style with a wider strap that had some padding underneath it. She learned to switch sides with her purse, sometimes wear it diagonally across her body, and not bear down on it when she was walking.

- At work, she adjusted her chair to fit her body so she could sit back in the seat. She raised her monitor (by putting it on a phone book) and lowered the keyboard. She was able to put the mouse at the same level as the keyboard and move it a lot closer. Throughout her workday, she became aware of the key concepts of balance, form, and perpetuating fluid flow.

For Tracy, the combination of these irritants would have accelerated the degenerative changes in her body in due time. With a few simple adjustments and some common sense, Tracy was instead able to reverse her pain and completely resolve her problems. She is now pain-free and happy to be so.

Although changing these habits can take a little time, it is certainly worth it in the long run.

IN THE POCKET

People, especially men, who do a lot of driving or sitting at work find that bulky items in their back pockets are a common source of irritation. Sure, it would be nice to have a huge wad of bills in your wallet, but such a windfall would only end up putting you out of balance. Billfolds, brushes, and receipt books carried in the back pocket can affect the balance in your hips, lower spine, lower back, and upper body. These items wedge underneath one hip and raise it to the side so there's an imbalance in the height of your hips relative to how you are sitting.

Instead of taking your wallet off your body, why not move it from a rear hip pocket to a front hip or shirt pocket? And try carrying your receipt books or brushes in a small briefcase or bag (or in the car). Remember,

How to Cough and Sneeze

A cough or a sneeze can be hazardous to your back health. This ordinary act of expelling air has been known to cause sharp, stabbing back pain. A simple technique can help ease the effect.

When you cough or sneeze, your body forces your diaphragm rapidly upward and contracts the abdominal muscles. This creates a burst of pressure to expel the foreign material or debris from your lungs. Just like an old tire will burst through at the weakest point, your cough or sneeze may find the path of least resistance. And sometimes that's your back.

If you have recently had abdominal surgery or have a weak area in your lower back because of a previous injury or strain, the additional forces will expand and stretch already weakened tissues and cause pain.

Here's the solution when you feel a cough or a sneeze coming on (assuming you aren't taken by surprise):

- Stand upright.
- Bend your knees rather deeply while keeping your body erect.
- Bend slightly forward with a hand on the mid-point of your thigh. This is for balance.
- Relax your abdominal muscles and your back muscles.
- Cover your mouth with your free hand, then cough or sneeze without forcefully flexing your head.
- Carefully return to the upright position.

Practice this technique to disperse the energy of a cough or sneeze. It really doesn't take as long to perform as it does to read.

though, that when you are changing a habit you've grown accustomed to (like moving your wallet to your shirt pocket), you have to be careful not to lose or misplace it.

GET A GRIP

There's a right and wrong way to grip what you carry. Grip too hard and you create unnecessary strain. Grip too softly, and you risk losing your grip. So, grip as tightly as needed to handle the load safely and without undue tension. Observe your hand and fingers as you move from any open position to a closed fist.

When you grip suitcases, briefcases, and other luggage, you also engage your hand muscles and slightly bent forearm to close your grip securely. You can make a firmer gripping surface by wrapping tape, gauze, or foam around the handle—a big help if you frequently have to grab on to and carry a particular bag.

Once you have a firm grasp, look at what the rest of your body is doing to move this load. Approach your suitcase or briefcase, bend your knees to lock in your balance, get a grip, use your legs, not back, and then stand upright. If you're carrying cases for a distance, think about packing two smaller ones to balance each other out, rather than one jumbo monster suitcase with everything you were afraid to leave home without.

If you'd rather get aerobic exercise some way other than lugging heavy cases, select luggage with rollers and pull/push handles that retract. Watch your body position while rolling or pushing them, to determine if you need to modify your posture or stop for a rest. Pushing a luggage cart seems to be easier for most people, but pulling your own bags with wheels works just fine as long as you hold your body in a forward position and don't twist and reach behind you. As in lifting, use your legs not your back, and don't jerk the suitcase. (You might want to rent a rolling cart, available at most airline luggage claim areas, or pay an attendant.)

17. HEALING AND REPAIRING AN INJURY

HEALING AND REPAIR IN TRUCKS AND HUMANS

Unlike the human body, a truck cannot rejuvenate itself. The best thing to do for a truck is to repair it as soon as damage or wear and tear becomes apparent. The earlier that any damage is detected in a truck's engine, frame, or electronics, the easier and more economical it is to fix, and the less likely it is that the damage will compound and begin to affect other parts of the truck.

A small patch of rust eventually grows and eats a hole in the body of the truck. The time to prevent that rust damage is when it first shows up—remove it immediately and then refinish the spot with quality automotive paint.

Black smoke emissions indicate there is something wrong with the fuel system. Blue smoke and gray smoke both indicate there is something wrong with the lubrication system. Whenever you find anything wrong in a truck, it is always advisable to fix it early, with quality parts. In the long run, you will save money and increase the longevity of the vehicle.

Wonders never cease when it comes to the human body because, unlike trucks, the body can heal and rejuvenate itself. A cut heals, a broken bone heals, and a sprained ankle heals. The only catch here is, these injuries don't always heal back to their original condition; they can leave scars, a limp, or a weak ankle, but, if appropriate treatment is applied early enough, you can increase your chances of eliminating any scars and limps. As with trucks, the earlier the treatment, the better the outcome—and the less pain and expense you will incur. Be sure, though, to continue treatment until you are fully functioning and your recovery is complete, not just

Mark's Story

While Mark was piloting an airplane, he got caught in a snowstorm and crashed, causing him to sustain extensive, life-threatening injuries. The force of the crash nearly ripped both his legs away at the knees, and, in addition, he had internal injuries, a broken jaw, a broken collarbone, and a concussion. Mark also had an incredible will to survive.

The emergency team tended first to his life-threatening injuries. They then set his collarbone, but several days later the orthopedic surgeons noticed that it had shifted. The broken bones were now overlapping by two inches. And they were healed. The doctors even considered rebreaking his bones and resetting them so they would mend in the proper position, but decided against it. They recommended instead that he learn to live with reduced function in his shoulders, or learn to do activities that would bring his shoulders back more toward their former position, and Mark opted for the latter choice. He understood, moreover, that this collarbone problem was relatively minor in comparison with his other injuries and with the long rehabilitation he needed to recover from knee and ligament transplants.

During his two years of intensive physical therapy, Mark could have chosen to recover just enough to hobble around and live a relatively mobile life. Instead, he chose the long, hard path to full recovery. He persevered and did what he had to do, despite the pain. Today, he plays volleyball, bikes, plays tennis, and has *few limits.* He knows his condition and knows what he needs to do each day to minimize the effects of his injuries.

---

until your pain is relieved. And don't let regrets rule the day, as they do with too many people, like the famous jazz musician, Eubie Blake, who ruefully said, "If I'd known I was going to live this long, I'd have taken better care of myself."

Never dismiss pain as "nothing" or as just an annoyance. Pain is your body's way of communicating that something is wrong. If left unattended, minor problems can quickly develop into major, chronic conditions. Look for and respond early to warning signs, such as numbness, pain, sleeplessness, stiffness, swelling, tingles, or undue fatigue. Seek the advice of a qualified healthcare provider for any minor problems or annoyances you may be having.

Treating minor problems early on increases your chances for a quick and complete recovery. And, as with trucks, maintaining your good health is instrumental to increasing your mileage.

RECOVERING FROM AN INJURY

When recovering from any injury, your primary intent is to heal the affected areas with optimum balance, form, and flow.

Time is also a factor in any full recovery, so keep it in mind as you recuperate. It can take six to twelve months to fully recover from a motor vehicle accident, for example. In the rehabilitation required for this, or for any recovery, daily repetition of the treatment and exercise programs makes all the difference.

18. FASHION STATEMENTS

PHYSICALLY FRIENDLY

Armed with a new perspective on how to evaluate and understand your physical environment, let's look at fashion and form. Those of us in health-care continually struggle with clothing issues. I personally believe the fashion world (the people who brought you platform shoes, lopsided haircuts, and tight jeans) has a great opportunity to bring aesthetically appealing and physically beneficial clothing into the world of fashion. Now all we have to do is get them on this bandwagon.

Clothing that does not fit your form can alter your balance and flow. Initially, ill-fitting apparel may seem inconsequential, and for the moment it is, but time will make even seemingly minor irritations and disruptions grow. From the perspective of balance, form, and flow, wearing less than ideally fitting clothes adversely affects and, slowly but surely, alters structure and function.

This is particularly important for children, as their growing bodies can be altered by the structural habits they develop in their formative years. Repetition compounds these numerous irritants for both children and adults because, if the items of apparel you carry or wear alter your movements in the transitions you make between walking, standing, and sitting in all your activities, the repetition of these altered movements will add to, and heighten, other irritants in your life.

IT'S IN THE JEANS

I frequently see what I call the jeans type of poor posture in pants that fit too tight and are too low in relation to a person's body type. These jeans can actually pull the lower back and hips backward when sitting, forcing a slump. It's difficult, even in an ideally fitting chair or car, to achieve a sound fit in these types of jeans.

The manner in which dresses, suits, pants, and coats are styled, and the way they hang on the body, directly impacts on how your form will alter your balance and movement. If the shoulder construction of a suit coat or overcoat does not fit the upper body and shoulders properly—if it's too loose for instance—you may end up thrusting your shoulders forward, or pulling your shoulders back, or keeping one shoulder up and out of balance, in order to hold the coat in position.

LOOSEN UP

Your blouses, dresses, jeans, and slacks can, over time, change their form and fit on your body. If people's clothes become too tight or too loose on them, it is common to see them struggling with those clothes, and altering their body positions to compensate for the ill fit.

Tight shirts, collars, ties, sweaters, or bras that constrict you can inhibit rib-cage movement and make it harder for you to maintain balance and have a balanced flow of oxygen. Belts, pants, skirts, and stockings can affect the function of the abdominal and back muscles and, in some cases, affect the function and fluid movement in your legs.

Watches, bracelets, and rings affect flow in the forearms and wrists, and can be a contributing factor in any strain or irritation you feel in those places. A too-tight watch or a bulky bracelet, for example, can impair your wrist action when you are keyboarding or using a calculator. Obviously, the solution is to remove them, but to do so, you first have to become aware of their harmful effects on your wrists.

IF YOUR SHOE FITS

Our feet are certainly our primary contact with the ground. They form the foundation for many of our upright postures and movements. If we didn't wear shoes regularly, the balance points of our feet would be (1) in the heel, (2) in the area underneath the knuckle of the big toe, and (3) across the arch to the side of the little toe.

In coordination with the arches, these contact points provide underlying support for the ankle, which then lays the groundwork for positioning of the knees, up through the upper leg and hips and into the upper back. This domino effect can be either stable and well-supported, or strained and distorted, with an imbalance in one causing an imbalance in all—serial distortion begins at the feet and works it way upward through the body.

It's critical for the contact positions of the feet and the integrity of the arches to be firmly aligned inside your shoes. Shoes fit if arch supports conform to the height and the width of the arch, and hold the foot in an appropriate position relative to the ankle. A shoe that is pointed or too narrow in the front can alter body balance and stability during walking, running, or standing in place.

The type of shoe worn can also vary according to your task, whether it is participating in such athletic activities as running, jumping, or walking, or attending business and social functions that do not require as much physical activity and exertion, but where fashion and function are still important.

Fluid flow can easily build up in your legs, particularly during periods of inactivity when you are sitting in one place, driving, or standing still. If you are wearing tight-fitting shoes, you can expect to have congested blood and lymphatic fluid in your toes or arches, or on the tops of the feet. You could also have swelling in your feet and lower legs, with increased tension in your calf and other leg muscles. Take these all as signals that your shoes are too tight.

DIFFERENT SOLES FOR DIFFERENT FOLKS

Athletic Shoes

Athletic shoes should be laced and tied to fit both your feet (for form and balance) and the athletic event, and they will vary depending on whether the event consists of standing, walking, jogging, running, jumping, moving straightforward or side to side (as in tennis or aerobic exercise), circular movements (like basketball), slow or fast movements, or a combination of all these.

Casual Shoes

Casual shoes should fit your form and balance as well as accommodate the length of time you are typically wearing them. The more time you spend wearing your shoes, the more important the incline of the sole and the type of cushion in the bottom of the shoe becomes. A sound cushion helps absorb the shock of standing on hard surfaces. If you intend to spend big bucks on shoes, spend them on the casual shoes you wear a lot.

Dress Shoes

Dress shoes should be comfortable and functional, plus match the fashion statement you wish to make. Remember, however, when choosing dress shoes it is smart, daring, and visionary to wear shoes that work for you *and* your feet.

OLD SHOES GIVE CLUES

Take a look at the shoes you wear most of the time and notice their wear patterns. The typical wear pattern may give you a clue what to look for in the next pair of shoes you buy. Where do your shoes wear out? In the toes? Heels? Wherever it is, that's where you need extra fortification.

Also look at the condition of your feet. You may discover what effects your shoes have had on your feet over time.

It is essential that shoes fit perfectly so use the following as guidelines to that end.

➤ In evaluating your shoes, determine whether they were designed for long-term (walking shoes) or short-term uses (the sequined heels that match the prom dress).

➤ Periodically examine the bottom of your shoes and their inside arches so you'll know when to have them either repaired or replaced.

➤ Next time you buy shoes, give them the wobble test: Put the shoes on a flat counter and see if they are solid or wobbly, or if one of them wobbles. This is what you're going to put on your feet. Is the sole curved? Too curved? Look for quality control here.

➤ Determine what types of repetitive movements you use while wearing certain shoes. If the shoe does not support the design of your foot during these movements, there can be undue strain or irritation inside the shoe, caused by seams opening, fabric buckling, or the arch and sole support lifting. This type of shifting can occur gradually, and the irritation that results can develop slowly, but many foot and ankle problems can be attributed to these changes occurring *inside* the shoe.

Martha's Story

Martha, a secretary for a large manufacturing company, was nearing retirement. She attributed her aches and pains to being sixty-one, but I discovered she had been heading for trouble for a long time simply because of the clothes she wore and the shoes she matched to them.

In the office where Martha worked, the accepted uniform included high-heeled shoes and rather tight, restrictive skirts that limited her mobility, especially when seated. I observed a domino effect here. The high heels she wore every day of her working life created ankle and lower leg problems, causing her to twist and distort her feet, in turn causing strain that traveled up her leg, through her knees (which tried to compensate), and eventually on up to her back. She had "taught" herself a new way to balance her body and it wasn't working very well for her.

Over the years, the heels, coupled with the tight clothing, had the effect of disturbing flow that changed her form. Had she only known this, she could have countered the cumulative injurious effects by stretching and doing exercises and movements designed to encourage positive outcomes.

Working together, however, we were gradually able to make things better for her by stretching her calf muscles, tendons, and feet enough to make them feel comfortable in flat shoes and allow her to finally walk barefoot at home for long periods of time. Through perseverance, Martha was able to reverse the effects of long-term wear and tear and return her body to a functionally younger form.

NEW HEIGHTS

The higher the heel of the shoe, of course, the more precarious your balance, not only for your foot and ankle, but also for your entire body. High heels trick your balancing mechanism into believing you are walking downhill because your ankle is inclined and your foot moves downward. Wearing high heels shortens the Achilles tendon, and constricts and contracts the calf and thigh muscles—all of which can also restrict fluid flow while, at the same time, forcing your whole body to pull slightly backward to remain erect or perpendicular with the ground.

This balancing act becomes even more tenuous when you attempt to move up and down stairs, walk on uneven ground, or simply stand. Each change of activity causes the body to go through the entire balancing cycle again and again. Not only are the muscles in your legs affected, but also the orientation of the hips, back, and shoulders relative to them is changed to some degree. And these factors are multiplied and magnified by time and repetition.

If you must wear high heels, special care should be taken to make sure the shoes have good arch support and do not crowd your feet. Give your feet a break, stretch your calf muscles, the Achilles tendon, and the arches of your feet regularly to counteract the accumulation of effects that occur with these types of shoes.

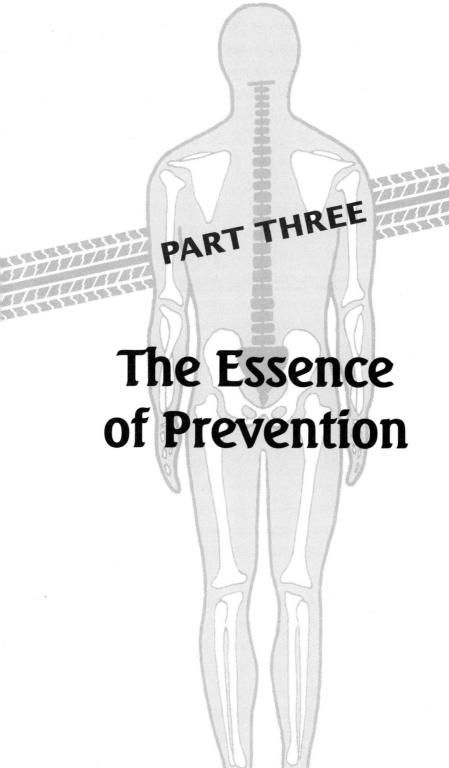

PART THREE

The Essence of Prevention

19. MAKING A DIFFERENCE

PREVENTIVE MEASURES IN TRUCKS AND HUMANS

A vehicle needs regular maintenance in all its systems—air, braking, electrical, fuel, lubrication, and so on. If you fail to maintain your truck, or allow it to become overworked and stressed, it is likely to fail you, and it can happen at any time, under any circumstances, exposing you and the truck to a higher risk of accidents. On the other hand, if you make sure your vehicle is well-maintained, it will be much more reliable, and therefore safer for you and all the others who share the road with you.

When it comes to the human body, illness and accident prevention also relies on maintenance. Maintaining a healthy diet, a regular exercise regimen, and regular sleeping habits gives you a nourishing lifestyle that will help you prevent accidents and limit excessive illness.

Also, for both trucks and humans, it is important to avoid dangerous circumstances, such as alcohol and drug abuse, which are leading factors in traffic accidents. They also, along with unsafe sex practices, are very deleterious to your overall health and well-being. In order to be well-maintained, for longevity, and to significantly decrease your chance of serious accidents and illness, you must keep yourself healthy, alert, and in control.

HOW TO CHANGE YOUR COURSE

How do you measure things that don't happen? For example, if you brush your teeth regularly, floss, use the right cavity-fighting toothpaste and the appropriate technique, get regular checkups, and heed the advice of your dentist, and you don't get cavities or gum disease, then you may be able to ascribe your good dental health to your regimen. But, can you measure if your regular exercise routine has prevented you from having a heart attack, or pushed the time you may eventually have a heart attack to much later in your life, or caused you to have a milder attack than you might otherwise have had? That's not as easy to do.

Preventive measures are difficult to quantify. That's why they're such a hard sell. You might even wonder if it's worth it to go through the prevention activities you do every day: brush your teeth, wear your safety belt, not smoke, choose a low-fat meal, walk, adjust your posture, and so on.

Since you may find it difficult to see the outcomes of your efforts, it's all the more important for you to understand why you do the things you do.

When it comes to balance and form and maintaining proper postures in daily activities, day after day, the outcome is clear—but difficult to pinpoint. You might be preventing pain and other aspects of physical aging, such as declining postures and degeneration. You could have less restriction in your movement and have fuller range of motion in your physical ability. You might even have added stamina. But you might have these attributes anyway as you age. Still, do you want to bet on it? What we *can* say with scientific certainty is that, if you don't respect your form and balance, your form and balance won't respect you, and you *will* suffer the consequences of aging.

Aging occurs slowly and over time, and it is the gradual aspect of this process that gives you the opportunity to intervene on your own behalf. You may not have any idea where and how these conditions are affecting your body, though sometimes you can see subtle changes, but it becomes clearer when you have had a chance to review your actions, habits, and behaviors.

ACCUMULATION

Imagine taking a handful of sand and letting the grains sift through your fingers onto the floor, then imagine that handful of sand being the individual stresses and strains throughout your day. You would be able to see the sand on the floor and it would be easy to sweep away and make the floor clean again.

If you swept up half the sand, the floor would look cleaner, but there would still be sand present. Suppose the next day you took another handful of sand and dropped it on the floor and again swept part of it away. If

Just Do It

I learned a lot about prevention the day I trimmed back the vines overgrowing the brick on our chimney. I had dreaded this task. The thought of precariously clinging to a ladder halfway up the side of the house was not my idea of a pleasant day of yard work. In fact, I had been avoiding it for weeks.

When I finished, I surveyed the newly bare brick and the four huge garbage bags filled with the vines that had threatened to take over like a little shop of horrors. Had I not waited so long to trim the vines, my task would have been easier by far. In fact, if I had gotten to this task in the springtime growing season, I could have redirected the thriving vines to become much fuller and healthier, and closer to their roots. Perhaps the vines would have lived a longer, fuller life had I taken better care of them earlier.

This story is not really about the vines growing on my house; that's just an analogy. I leave it to you to make your own "gardening" agenda so *your* "vines" can flourish and have a long, full life. Start sowing the seeds now.

—Dr. Scott W. Donkin

you were to continue like this, dropping grains of sand on your floor, day after day, for a long period of time, and only sweeping up part of the pile, sand would accumulate, and, in time, you would have created a very noticeable mound. Now imagine all this sand being the individual stresses and strains that assault you throughout the day and you can see how they can accumulate if not swept away.

Just as prevention can help you sweep away all the grains of sand every day, so, too, can you sweep away the accumulation of strains and tensions that accelerate the aging process. You can replace them by caring for your body every day through smart body management, relaxation, and improving your balance, form, and flow. The result of your preventive actions will be a collectively improved state of health and well-being.

ACCELERATORS OF CHANGE

Time, repetition, and other factors cause the momentum for a change that can be either positive or negative for you. Here are some key factors to keep in mind as you decide whether you want to accelerate change for the better or not:

➤ First, know that your attitude and consistency toward action or inaction are primary key factors in this decision.

➤ Live in the present, but understand that everything you do in the present affects your future—your destiny—so keep your eyes and your actions on the long-term goals.

➤ Create change faster by being aware of the activities that encompass the larger parts of your day, and make changes based on that awareness.

➤ Accelerate change by repetition of your actions and habits.

➤ Use vibration and appropriate sound frequencies, forms of repetition (sound), to change your balance, flow, and form.

➤ Recognize that relaxation and the process of internally letting changes happen are essential.

My Personal Change

At forty, I was a workaholic, rushing and abusing my health with a stressful, obsessive sense of duty. I frequently drank coffee and alcohol, ate unhealthy food, smoked a lot, and did nothing more than complain about my aching body.

One day, I recognized that my behaviors were causing my problem, and I realized I could change how I felt by altering my negative behaviors.

Today, I am fifty-plus years young and still growing. I don't feel any further need to smoke, or drink caffeine or alcohol. I eat healthy food and I enjoy life. You can too!

—Gérard Meyer

20. TOTAL BODY MANAGEMENT

CLEANING AND CARE IN TRUCKS AND HUMANS

Professional trucking companies understand the importance of regularly cleaning trucks. A clean truck is a sign of a well-run, successful company and adds to its efficiency and longevity.

Cleaning a truck involves more than washing its windows, body, and mirrors, and throwing away trash that has accumulated during a long haul. It also means flushing the radiator periodically, changing the oil, its filter, and other filters and fluids, which all enhance the performance of the truck. Additionally, a truck is more protected and runs more efficiently if it is cleaned before greasing and relubricating. A thoroughly clean truck, inside and out, runs better and looks better to its owners, its driver, and the rest of the world.

Similarly, many people view a clean person as an outward sign of professionalism, competence, and success. Cleaning a human body includes more than daily personal hygiene and baths or showers. Cleaning the inside of a human body is of the utmost importance in maintaining good health and vigor. This includes proper waste elimination to rid the body of the impurities and toxins that accumulate in our systems as a matter of course.

Water, exercise, and stretching are the prime ways to assist your body in its efforts to keep the inside clean. As previously discussed, water is the essential fluid in all the body's systems, including digestion and elimination. Even muscles are largely made up of water (75 percent). Regular exercise and muscle stretching increases the flow of blood, the lymphatic fluids, and the air to the lungs. All are important in maintaining optimum flow, as well as cleansing your body.

When your body is clean on the inside, you'll have more efficient operation of all its systems: central nervous, circulatory, lymphatic, and digestive. And with all these systems in peak performance, you'll be less likely to develop illnesses and injury.

FUEL AND NUTRITION IN TRUCKS AND HUMANS

The two basic concerns that truck owners have about fuel are engine longevity and fuel conservation. Putting unleaded gas in a diesel engine would have the immediate negative consequence of engine failure. And what would happen if you poured sugar or flour into a truck's fuel tank? Again, engine failure. Proper fuel is crucial to maximal engine performance.

Fuel consumption can be reduced by 20 percent or more if a driver uses a sensible driving style, if the truck has had regular and complete maintenance, and if it receives the right kind of fuel.

Food is to the human body what fuel is to trucks, and the type of food you eat has a profound effect on your body's form and functioning. Healthy food promotes well-being and longevity, as well as mental alertness and stamina.

Nutrition is, in fact, fundamental to achieving overall health and living a long life. And the quality of that nutrition (plus the other essential life forces that are flowing through your body) is extremely important to your physical health and longevity if you want to live free of the degenerative diseases that plague too many older people. Exactly what is important and how much is important is controversial. Volumes have been written on nutrition and continual research advances our knowledge of it.

It is also vital to supplement your intake of nutrients with sufficient pure water, at least eight glasses a day. Putting enough water into your system is essential to the flow of fluids in your body, in order for them to eliminate waste, cleanse tissues, and transport nutrients. If this fluid flow is disturbed, even with a proper intake of nutrients, your tissues can't get what they need. More than once, I've seen chronically tight back or leg muscles, the result of injuries that have not healed properly. Because of the high percentage of water in muscles, they need water to function properly, but with the flow impaired by lack of water, these tissues cannot get the nutrients they need for proper healing. In every case I've treated, the chronic tightness has vanished after my advice to drink lots of high quality water has been followed.

FOOD GUIDE PYRAMID

The U.S. Department of Health and Human Services has devised a helpful food pyramid. If you follow its guidelines for food, you will be going a long way toward promoting good health and helping your body maintain a fit form.

FOOD PYRAMID (Inverted)

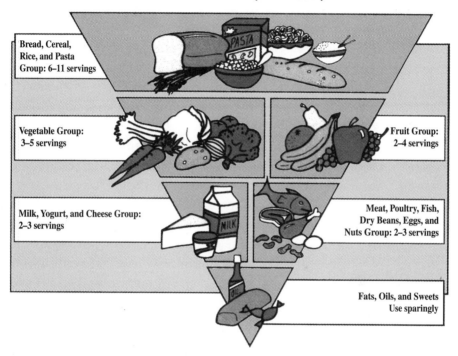

Bread, Cereal, Rice, and Pasta Group: 6–11 servings

Vegetable Group: 3–5 servings

Fruit Group: 2–4 servings

Milk, Yogurt, and Cheese Group: 2–3 servings

Meat, Poultry, Fish, Dry Beans, Eggs, and Nuts Group: 2–3 servings

Fats, Oils, and Sweets Use sparingly

You'll notice the serving quantities decrease as we go down the list. That's why it's called an inverted pyramid. You should consume fewer servings that are listed at the bottom, and center your diet on the groups at the top, selecting nonfat and lean foods as often as possible.

VISION AND EYE CARE IN TRUCK DRIVING AND HUMAN DRIVING

What a nightmare it would be to drive a truck and not be able to see out the windows. You, and all around you, would be put at risk. Obviously, an unhampered sight line is essential to controlling the vehicle and preventing accidents. Windows should be cleaned, inside and out, on a regular basis.

They should be free of cracks and chips. Mirrors should also give you clear vision. Headlights should be free of dirt and debris in order to give you maximum illumination for night driving.

The interior of the truck should provide you with enough good light to read maps or documents. The instruments should be clearly visible at all times, not obstructed or dirty. Defrosters should be kept in topnotch shape for those wintry and rainy days. Windshield wipers must be pliable and reliable.

It is also important for all reflectors, taillights, and running lights to be in good working order so other drivers can clearly see you. Again, regular maintenance and repair of all these keeps your view of the instruments and the road clear, and helps you prevent accidents (an estimated 25 percent of all motor vehicle accidents are attributed at least in part to visual impairments).

What beautiful eyes you have. If you want to keep your vision as good as your eyes are beautiful, then regular eye care is extremely important, and often overlooked. Heredity, age, eyestrain, and nutrition have a lot to do with the degeneration of eyes, but you can maintain your eyesight by having regular checkups and by alternately resting and exercising your eyes.

A qualified eye professional should immediately check any vision disturbance you might experience. Some vision problems are symptoms of diabetes or high blood pressure, or other serious health issues. Some vision problems can be caused by allergic reactions or overdosing on drugs or medications. That is why it is important to have your eyes checked and find the cause of your problem early so the treatment you are given has a better chance of succeeding.

Looking at a fixed distance for long periods of time, at a computer monitor, or down a long highway can cause eye fatigue. If your eye muscles are strained, your concentration will be disrupted and that will affect your job performance and well-being.

To minimize this strain, you need to give your eyes frequent vision breaks. This means that you should frequently change your depth of vision, looking from near to far and back. This helps exercise and maintain flexibility of the lens and the eyes.

Another good set of eye exercises is as follows:

1. Roll your eyes in a circle, both clockwise and counterclockwise;

2. Move them as far right and then as far left as you can;

3. Next, look up as high as possible and then down as low as possible;

4. Last, move your eyes up and down diagonally, top left to bottom right, and vice versa.

These exercises work the muscles that move the eyes, and you should try to do them as often as you can. I recommend at least a hundred times for each. This may seem like a lot, but they can be done anywhere, while walking, sitting, standing in an elevator, waiting for a green light, an appointment, etc., and they do work. The movement helps lubricate the eyes, and also eases tension in the muscles, besides giving the skin around your eyes a good workout.

EXERCISE

There is no question that exercise is an absolutely fundamental element of structural longevity. Among other things, appropriate aerobic and flexibility exercise reduces the onset and severity of osteoporosis, neutralizes the negative effects of stress, and produces a sense of accomplishment and happiness.

With any exercise program, you can also evaluate its importance and effectiveness by making sure to consider the following:

Balance

Does your exercise provide movements you need for the full range of motion you do not get during the day or night? Specifically, does your regimen give you back and upper-body extension to counteract the typical forward-oriented movements and postures?

Form

Does your exercise work to improve your physical condition, your stamina, and your muscle and ligament balance, and does it function in accordance with your own physical makeup? Does it encourage stretching, breathing, mental relaxation, and clarity?

Flow

Does your regimen stimulate the flow of air, fluids, and body movements to all parts of your body, especially to those that receive less flow during the day or night as a result of your unique set of habits?

Time

Does your exercise occur with enough time and repetition to create, continue, or accelerate the changes in balance, form, and flow that you want?

Repetition

Do you repeat the beneficial moves that help you ingrain positive habits into your body often enough?

WHAT ARE YOU GOING TO DO NOW?

As a society, we have made better things, but somewhere we have lost touch with how to make things better for ourselves and others. We have paid for losing touch with our simpler but very real needs over the last several generations (and maybe even longer).

As has always been the case, real change and transformation is well within our grasp and can, in many respects, occur as quickly as changing our minds. From this point in time, to achieve maximum benefit, it is important for you to study yourself:

➤ Review the figures and the key points that seemed most meaningful for you in this book.

➤ Look at your balance in a nonjudgmental fashion. Observe your habits, what you've been doing through the course of your day, day after day, when you've lost touch with your conscious physical activities while you've been thinking of other things. Look at the accumulation of your habits to this point.

➤ Look at pictures of yourself and ask others around you for input and insight.

➤ Review your actions and habits and determine the course you are presently on. If you continue to do the things you are doing, where are you going to end up?

➤ Where are you now? Where do you want to be?

After you have made these determinations, you can pull away from your daily habits and look objectively at them. Change the things you can. You don't have to change everything at once. Small changes build momentum. Remember, *repetition and time have the effect of changing balance, form, and flow*. You can actually alter your destiny.

At this point, it would be a good idea to refer to the Self-Evaluation Test in Appendix A. Wherever you have a low score on any of the 8 steps, you should devote more time to those sections of the book that deal with the possible solutions for your circumstances. If you are having difficulty making changes in one area, don't stop, don't give up. Go to a different area and work on those. Nothing is going to change unless you take the first step, then the next, and the next.

The stress reaction can negate your efforts, so remember not to be too anxious or harsh on yourself. Don't allow the stress reaction to work against you.

You cannot make any changes unless you wake up to the fact that you need to make them and they might be beneficial for you. By the same token, once you realize you must make changes, you can determine how these enhancements will positively benefit you.

If it is difficult for you to arrive at that firm decision to make major changes at this time, then try a few key changes and see if you can feel your way into changing other things. Keep your destiny in mind, and, along the way, enjoy the benefits of your changes.

As you are going through this process, you will undoubtedly experience numerous successes and have many insights into solving a problem—something that has been perhaps tormenting you, or has become a continuous source of irritation that you didn't even know about, at least consciously. When you finally resolve it, it can become quite exciting.

What if you end up living a longer life than you expect? Looking back, if you had only made subtle changes allowing time and repetition to work for you, you would have experienced profound positive changes in your destiny. Fortunately, you're at a point where you don't have to look back with regret, you can make changes now so you *will* experience profound changes in your destiny.

If in doubt about what you should do relative to your unique circumstances, by all means seek the assistance of experts and your healthcare professionals so you don't do anything that could be a problem for you.

CONCLUSION

IF THE SHOE FITS, WHY DOESN'T EVERYTHING ELSE?

You don't have to be "young at heart" to live to 105. You need to be structurally sound so that when you reach a healthy old age, your body is there to support you. Yet Americans suffer from a personal crumbling infrastructure—not our bridges or highways, but our bones and muscles, backs and joints.

Like a left shoe on the right foot, we've been trying to shoehorn our bodies into the wrong shoes and causing ourselves unnecessary and painful wear and tear in the process. We have been:

➤ Sitting in the wrong-sized chairs at work and loungers at home;

➤ Reaching over poorly fitting workstations;

➤ Crunching into cars that are too small or too big;

➤ Jackknifing into uncomfortable restaurant booths and awkward patio furniture;

➤ Slumping in front of computer screens, especially laptops, that are at the wrong level;

➤ Grabbing telephones that are too far away;

➤ Standing in line, leaning over a grocery cart;

➤ Sleeping in hotel beds that are too soft or too hard, or in our own beds with pillows that take the rest out of sleep;

➤ Crouching in airline seats where one size fits nobody;

➤ Gardening, sweeping, vacuuming, and washing the car in awkward positions;

➤ Reading in bed and watching a TV that's improperly positioned;

➤ Lifting, and paying the price with back pain later;

➤ Carrying all kinds of items improperly, including purses, luggage, back-packs, and briefcases; and

➤ Purchasing and wearing clothing that puts our bodies in the "wrong shoe."

If the shoe fits, why doesn't everything else? You can now make the difference for yourself and feel better, plus reduce or prevent much misery in your future.

APPENDIX A

PEAK PERFORMANCE
SELF-EVALUATION TEST

Eight Steps to Achieving
Peak Performance Body and Mind

To take this short test, please read each statement and indicate your first response to it with the abbreviations below. We suggest you use a separate sheet of paper and take this test at one- to six-month intervals so you can see the effects of the changes you are making in your life. Be sure to date your score sheets and keep them for future reference. Also, check our website www.peakhealthandsafety.com for updated versions of this test and its scoring.

Strongly Agree	SA
Agree	A
Undecided	U
Disagree	D
Strongly Disagree	SD

STEP 1

A. Mental Concept of Age   SA   A   U   D   SD

I usually feel much younger than my age.

B. Influence the Future   SA   A   U   D   SD

The habits I have and the actions I take determine the quality of
my health and well-being in the future.

STEP 2

C. Flexibility of Upper Body   SA   A   U   D   SD

I can look over my right and left shoulder without twisting
my body, and see clearly to back up in my vehicle.

D. Flexibility of Lower Body   SA   A   U   D   SD

I can bend over to touch my toes without pain or stiffness,
and I can lean backward without pain or stiffness.

**E. Flexibility and Activities
of Daily Living**   SA   A   U   D   SD

I can put on my underwear and socks and tie my shoes
without any pain or stiffness.

F. Breathing   SA   A   U   D   SD

I frequently take time during the day to sit or stand upright,
breathe in deeply, and exhale slowly and completely.

STEP 3

G. Time   SA   A   U   D   SD

I usually have enough time to do what I want and need to do.

H. Outlook on Life   SA   A   U   D   SD

I will do the things I believe will help me be as healthy
as possible because I will be healthier over the course
of my life, and I expect to live a long life.

I. Self-Assessment of Life   SA   A   U   D   SD

I believe I have accomplished a lot in my life so far
and I am pleased at this point.

J. Time and Aging   SA   A   U   D   SD

Time has very little to do with the quality of the
aging process.

STEP 4

K. Energy   SA   A   U   D   SD

I have more than enough energy to do all of
my daily activities.

L. Flexibility, Strength, and Stamina   SA   A   U   D   SD

I have more flexibility, strength, and stamina
than I had three months ago.

M. Outlook on Situations   SA   A   U   D   SD

I always find the bright side of a situation.

STEP 5

N. Reaction to Stressors   SA   A   U   D   SD

When I encounter stressful situations, I usually
deal with them to the best of my ability and
resolve them in my mind.

O. Stress Management   SA   A   U   D   SD

I usually resolve stressful situations and take care
of myself so they do not cause me to be physically
tense or mentally drained.

P. Worry   SA   A   U   D   SD

I do not usually let worry affect me physically
or mentally.

STEP 6

Q. Sitting   SA   A   U   D   SD

I can sit comfortably for as long as I want in my
chair or vehicle because I know how to sit, and
also how to keep pressure and tension from
building up in my body.

R. Standing   SA   A   U   D   SD

I can stand comfortably for as long as I want
because I know how to relieve the buildup of
pressure or tension in my body.

S. Activities   SA   A   U   D   SD

I spend at least 30 minutes every day doing
health-improving activities, such as exercising,
stretching, reading positive books, listening
to positive tapes, etc.

T. Fatigue   SA   A   U   D   SD

I can drive, work, or read comfortably for as long
as I want without becoming tired or fatigued.

STEP 7

U. Quality of Rest and Alertness   SA   A   U   D   SD

I never take medication like pain pills, muscle
relaxers, sleeping pills, or stimulants.

V. Quality of Waking Up   SA   A   U   D   SD

I usually wake up refreshed after sleeping, and
look forward to the day ahead of me.

W. Sleeping Comfort   SA   A   U   D   SD

I can sleep comfortably through the night
without pain or stiffness.

STEP 8

X. Water   SA   A   U   D   SD

I drink at least eight 8 oz. glasses of water a day.

Y. Eating   SA   A   U   D   SD

I know the foods I should be eating and almost
always eat them.

Z. Tobacco, Alcohol, and Caffeine   SA   A   U   D   SD

I use alcohol and caffeine in moderation and
never use tobacco.

SCORES:

Score your own test by giving yourself the following points for each of
your responses:

Strongly Agree (SA)	5 Points
Agree (A)	4 Points
Undecided (U)	3 Points
Disagree (D)	2 Points
Strongly Disagree (SD)	1 Point

In this simple scoring system, the higher the score the better. A response
of SA or A is good while a score of D or SD suggests that you should
look at the corresponding section of the book to help you improve your
score and, more important, improve the quality of your life *one step at a
time.* Steps 1–8 are explained below.

Maximum Score: 130 Points

110–130   AWESOME. You probably have many good habits that will
serve you well now and in the future. Read this book to keep
yourself on track.

90–110   GOOD. You have a number of good habits and you would benefit from learning what activities and beliefs are helping you, as well as discovering those you can improve on.

60–90   FAIR. There are probably several sections of this book you should concentrate on to improve your state of health and well-being.

26–60   TIME TO CHANGE. You have made a wise choice to study this book. Learn which unwise habits you have. It is very important for you to become aware of the improvements you can make in your life now because you probably won't like the end result of the body/mind path you are presently on.

Step 1—Pain and Acceptance of Aging

Believing that you can influence your health and well-being through your habits is critical to gaining maximum benefit from this book. Take a closer look at the Introduction, as well as Chapters 1, 2, and 3 to help you here.

Step 2—Mobility and Flexibility

Seemingly minor changes in your flexibility actually chart your course toward peak health or gradual breakdown. It is essential to regularly be aware of your body's optimum movement patterns and habits. Chapters 2, 4, and 6 will, therefore, be important for you to understand.

Step 3—Time Management

Improving your understanding of time, coupled with learning how to take advantage of time, usually determines your level of success in achieving peak performance. Focus on Chapters 5 and 8 to help you here.

Step 4—Energy Level and Stamina

It is nearly impossible to achieve and maintain better habits without quality rest and good energy levels. Concentrate on Chapters 7 and 14 for this. Also, our website www.peakhealthandsafety.com will help you greatly here.

Step 5—Stressor Identification

Stressors come at us from many directions, some of which we recognize, most of which we don't. To gain more awareness of how stress affects you, in order to better control it, spend some extra time on Chapter 9.

Step 6—Poor Habits and Discomfort

These habits will make or break the quality of your health and well-being over time. To better manage these habits, look to Chapters 10, 11, 12, 13, 15, 16, and 18.

Step 7—Quality and Quantity of Rest and Alertness

How you rest and sleep, as well as how you maintain alertness, all have a profound impact on your motivation to either work regularly to improve yourself and your surroundings, or just let your health and well-being slip away. The information and tips in Chapter 14 will help you here.

Step 8—Intake and Dependencies

The positive and negative effects of substances you put into your body, especially on a regular basis, directly affect the health of your body and your mind. Here, it is very important to become aware of the pivotal impact your intake has so you can make informed decisions on how to balance it, and not be driven only by your habits. Read Chapter 20, and access our website www.peakhealthandsafety.com for more valuable information.

Appendix B

Corporate and Individual Solutions

As you read through the chapters in this book, you will become more aware of yourself and your surroundings. You will also undoubtedly discover aspects of your environment, such as automobile seats, beds, pillows, chairs, and clothing, to name a few, that do not fit you properly, so you may want to contact us for individual questions or help.

Like individuals, companies frequently have challenges with health and safety issues affecting their employees. Also, just as individuals who do not pay attention to their habits will not usually enjoy a peak-performance life, companies that do not pay attention to employee health and safety circumstances will not enjoy peak corporate performance and profitability. Corporate needs are best assessed and dealt with using a variety of products and services, including the ones we offer.

Whether you have individual or corporate needs, you can contact us at our website www.peakhealthandsafety.com. You can also call our message and order center at 1-800-552-6347 (U.S. only) to ask questions or request information. Here are a few of the services and products that can help both individuals and companies.

SERVICES

All services described below can be accessed through our website.

➤ We have developed a remarkable CLOSED-LOOP COMPUTER-BASED TRAINING PROGRAM to accelerate the learning process outlined in this book, and it is designed to automatically adjust to your own pace.

➤ BIONOMICS is a new term developed through Future Industrial Technologies by its president, Dennis Downing. It is a field related to ergonomics that combines the teaching of biomechanics, posture, and non-strenuous stretching. The goal of Bionomics is to teach, through proper body management, how to prevent the occurrence of physical stress in the first place or, if there is already physical stress present, how to relieve the body of any accumulation of it. This training, known as *BACKSAFE™* and *SITTINGSAFE™*, is performed in small group settings conducted by one of more than 1,100 trained facilitators throughout North America. If companies comply with the recommendations made during the initial assessment and the subsequent phases of the program, they can usually reduce the incidence and/or cost of work injuries by 40 to 70 percent. Participants learn how to be responsible for their own physical well-being, both on and off the job. *BACKSAFE* and *SITTINGSAFE* training both complement the information in this book, and both are excellent ways to effectively transform your habits with professional guidance.

➤ THE INDUSTRIAL ATHLETE PROGRAM™ was conceived and developed by Drs. Allen and Jennifer Miller, originally in response to rising workers compensation claims. Both doctors had worked in the fields of Olympic and Professional sports, helping to treat athletes' injuries and improve their performance. In these fields, computerized methods for testing athletes' physical abilities were common. When they shifted to a general practice, however, they discovered that those techniques for evaluating and treating injuries were not available to the workforce, so they developed a program based upon the athletic model to meet this need. The workplace has benefited greatly from this program, which has succeeded in reducing costs, providing better treatment, and increasing companies' profitability.

➤ Dr. Brock Walker's ENGINEERED SEATING SOLUTIONS will soon be available in several user-friendly forms for all parts of our lives. Dr. Walker is an expert in enhancing human performance and successfully treating musculoskeletal problems. After a series of personal injuries, he turned to designing seating, and his research and engineering solutions have already been used in the aerospace and motorsports industries. One of his most successful solutions was for Buddy Lazier after a serious accident in 1996 had left the race-car driver with multiple spinal fractures and unable to stand, sit, or lay down without experiencing excruciating pain. The safe, supportive seat that Dr. Walker designed for Buddy's race car allowed him to compete in, and WIN, the grueling Indianapolis 500. If Dr. Walker can ameliorate such a dire condition, imagine what he can do for the rest of us.

➤ We offer CORPORATE HEALTH AND SAFETY MANAGEMENT, and can customize solutions for you based on our analysis of the needs and risks involved We work with several organizations, including the ACA Council on Occupational Health, and the related IACOHC, that can offer additional solutions.

➤ Our MOTIVATIONAL WORKSHOPS AND SEMINARS, based on our unique and prevention-oriented concepts, are specifically designed to achieve practical results.

➤ For personal and corporate applications, we can EVALUATE AN INDI-VIDUAL'S PHYSICAL CAPACITY AND PERFORMANCE using high-tech methods.

➤ The subject was beyond the scope of our first book, but we have now made information available on PROPER NUTRITION, SUPPLEMENTA-TION, AND WATER, which are essential components for a peak per-formance body and mind.

PRODUCTS

All products and guidelines below can be accessed through our website.

➤ The *BACK FLEX*™ HEALTHY BACK SYSTEM is an innovative method for relieving back strain while improving posture. Regular use can relieve back pain, slumping, and stress, and can increase the users' awareness of how to adjust their own chairs, desks, seats, etc. to fit better for good posture.

➤ We can provide CD-ROM-BASED INTERACTIVE VIDEO PROGRAMS ON HEALTH AND SAFETY. The routines are specifically designed for improved balance, flexibility, posture, strength, and stress manage-ment. These kits also include printed material, Swiss exercise balls or exercise tubing, and are very user-friendly and portable.

➤ INNOVATIVE CUSHIONS, PILLOWS, SUPPORTS, AND WEDGES are available here or through links we can provide to other sources. Made from a variety of materials, all are designed to help match your unique form and needs to your environment and the tasks you perform.

➤ We have GUIDELINES FOR PURCHASING everything from clothing to vehicles, which are based on how well the item would fit in terms of its function, fashion, and value.

References

American Heritage Dictionary. Boston, MA: Houghton Mifflin Company, 1992.

Bagot, Jean-Didier. *Information, Sensation et Perception.* Paris, France: Armand Colin, 1999.

Berthoz, A. *Le Sens du Mouvement.* Paris, France: Editions Odile Jacob, 1995.

Boyd, William. *Textbook of Pathology,* 8th Edition. Philadelphia, PA: Lea, Febiger, 1970.

Brannon, Linda, Jess Feist. *Health Psychology: An Introduction to Behavior and Health.* Belmont, CA: Wadsworth/Thomson Learning, 2000.

Camus, Jean-Francois. *La Psychologie Cognitive de l'Attention.* Paris, France: Armand Colin, 1996.

Donkin, Scott. *Sitting on the Job.* North Bergen, NJ: Basic Health Publications, 2002.

Grandjean, E. *Fitting the Task to the Man.* Philadelphia, PA: Taylor & Francis, Ltd, 1985.

Grandjean, E. *Ergonomics of the Home.* Philadelphia, PA: Taylor & Francis, Ltd, 1978.

Gray, H. *Gray's Anatomy.* Philadelphia, PA: Running Press, July 1999.

Guyton, Arthur C. *Guyton Physiology.* Philadelphia, PA: W.B. Saunders, 2000.

Junghanns, H. *Clinical Implications of Normal Biomechanical Stress on Spinal Function.* Gaithersburg, MD: Aspen Publishers, Inc., 1990.

Harrison, D, et al. Chiropractic Biophysics Technique: A Linear Algebra Approach to Posture in Chiropractic. *Journal of Manipulative and Physiological Therapeutics* 19 no. 8 (October 1996):525–535.

Harrison, D, et al. Comparisions of Lordotic Cervical Spine Curvatures to a Theoretical Ideal Model of the Static Sagittal Cervical Spine. *Journal of Manipulative and Physiological Therapeutics* 21 no. 6 (March 1996):667–675.

Harrison, D, et al. Elliptical Modeling of the Sagittal Lumbar Lordosis and Segmental Rotation Angles as a Method to Discriminate Between Normal and Low Back Pain Subjects. *Journal of Spinal Disorders* 11 no. 5 (March 1998):1–10.

Isernhagen, S. *Work Injury: Management and Prevention.* Gaithersburg, MD: Aspen Publishers, Inc. 1988.

Kreiger, C. *Posture and Pain.* New York, NY: Kendall and Kendall, 1985.

Laville, A. *L'Ergonomie, Le Point des Connaissances Actuelles.* Paris, France: Puf, 1998.

Monod, H., Kapitaniak, B. *Ergonomie.* Paris, France: Masson, 1999.

Pheasant, S. *Ergonomics, Work and Health.* Gaithersburg, MD: Aspen Publishers, Inc., 1991.

Sorsana, C. *Psychologie des Interactions Sociocognitives.* Paris, France: Armand Colin, 1999.

Stedman, T. *Stedman's Medical Dictionary,* 26th ed. Baltimore, MD: Williams & Wilkins, 1995.

Twerski, A. *Addictive Thinking: Understanding Self-Deception.* Center City, MN: Hazelden Foundation, 1990.

Whang, S. *Reverse Aging.* Englewood Cliffs, NJ: Siloam Enterprise, Inc., 1994.

Williams, L. *Teaching for the Two-Sided Mind.* New York, NY: A Touchstone Book. Simon & Schuster, Inc., 1986.

Witten, M, Vincent, D. *Computational Medicine, Public Health, and Biotechnology, Part II.* London, England: World Scientific Publishing Co., Pte, Ltd, 1994.

INDEX

ABOUT THE
AUTHORS

DR. SCOTT W. DONKIN, DC, DACBOH

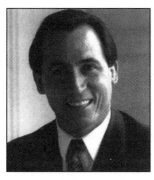

Dr. Donkin is an internationally published author, chiropractor, lecturer, and consultant who has been in private practice in Lincoln, Nebraska, for twenty years.

His classic work, *Sitting on the Job,* published in Britain as *Fit for Work,* broke new ground by addressing the needs of the seated workplace and helping to transform poor sitting behaviors while increasing workers' efficiency and pre-venting injuries. In line with helping people develop better habits and better health, Dr. Donkin has also produced numerous multimedia programs on CDs, audiocassettes, videos, and slides.

Dr. Donkin has written for numerous professional journals, and inter-views with him have appeared in popular magazines, such as *Conde Nast Traveler, Inc.,* and *Self,* and newspapers, including *The Wall Street Journal* and *The Los Angeles Times.* He has also been a frequent guest on radio and tele-vision talk shows.

He lectures and consults throughout North America on human per-formance, ergonomics, health, and wellness for corporations, organiza-tions, and government agencies. He has evaluated airplane seats and hotel mattresses for *USA Today,* and has consulted widely on workplace modifi-cations, determining specifications and evaluating products for workplace acquisitions.

He is a member and former president of the American Chiropractic

Association Council on Occupational Health, and a member of the Medical Advisory Board for The Wellness Councils of America, as well as for its publication, *Healthy YOUniverse.*

Dr. Donkin graduated from Texas Chiropractic College in Pasadena, Texas. He had postgraduate training in orthopedics, industrial consulting, and ergonomics, and is a Board Certified Diplomate of the American Chiropractic Board of Occupational Health.

DR. GÉRARD MEYER

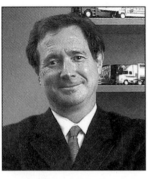

Dr. Gérard Meyer was born and educated in France where he studied industrial safety, engineering, and psychology as an undergraduate. He received his doctorate in Ergonomic Physiology and was appointed Chief Advisor to the French Minister for Technical Education where he oversaw all the agency's international and cooperative development between France and the United States.

Dr. Meyer is the founder and former president and CEO of the Carnegie Mellon Driver Training and Safety Institute (CM-DTSI) in the United States. He heads an international team of industry experts and top researchers who are identifying and selecting the most advanced, effective, educational methods to train drivers in safety and productivity. He has coordinated a partnership between government, education, industry, and community agencies to research, develop, and implement these programs.

Dr. Meyer has also organized a transatlantic consortium for vocational training, which includes the United States, Denmark, Sweden, The Netherlands, and other European countries. Its purpose is to exchange information, research, and technology that will lead to better training, health, and safety for drivers throughout Europe and the United States. Dr. Meyer currently resides in Pittsburgh, Pennsylvania.